METHODS IN MEDICINE

METHODS IN MEDICINE

A Descriptive Study of Physicians' Behaviour

J. RIDDERIKHOFF

Department of Family Medicine, Erasmus University,
Rotterdam, the Netherlands

KLUWER ACADEMIC PUBLISHERS
DORDRECHT / BOSTON / LONDON

Library of Congress Cataloging in Publication Data

Ridderikhoff, J., 1932-
   Methods in medicine : a descriptive study of physicians' behaviour
/ J. Ridderikhoff.
      p.   cm.
   Bibliography: p.
   Includes index.
   ISBN 1-556-08080-8
   1. Physicians--Psychology. 2. Problem-solving. 3. Decision
-making. 4. Medicine--Practice--Psychological aspects.   I. Title.
   [DNLM: 1. Behavior. 2. Physicians--psychology. 3. Professional
Practice.   W 87 R543m]
   R690.R53 1989
   610.69'52'019--dc19
   DNLM/DLC
   for Library of Congress   88-12961
                                                                  CIP

Published by Kluwer Academic Publishers,
P.O. Box 17, 3300 AA Dordrecht, The Netherlands

Kluwer Academic Publishers incorporates
the publishing programmes of
D. Reidel, Martinus Nijhoff, Dr W. Junk and MTP Press.

Sold and distributed in the U.S.A. and Canada
by Kluwer Academic Publishers,
101 Philip Drive, Norwell, MA 02061, U.S.A.

In all other countries, sold and distributed
by Kluwer Academic Publishers Group,
P.O. Box 322, 3300 AH Dordrecht, The Netherlands.

Printed in the Netherlands

Dedicated to my wife,
Diny, my two sons, Hans and Paul,
and particularly to my parents,
without whose creation this book would
never have been born.

Contents

Preface

Clinicians spend their working lives making decisions. such decisions are usually made in interlocking streams rather than in the discrete circumscribed contexts so beloved of scientists. When the clinician encounters a patient a complex interactive process is initiated in which the clinician searches his memory to match the symptoms and signs indicated by the patient with the complex disease models which he carries in his head. He then makes choices about further questions or tests in order to clarify his understanding of the patient's problem and to formulate a management or treatment plan. In recent years there has been increasing interest in how clinicians make such decisions and a realization that decision-making in clinical medicine is virtually the same as that in many other professional contexts.

The scientific study and formal teaching of clinical decision-making is a relatively young discipline. Less than 20 books have so far appeared which take explicit account of the theoretical and experimental decision-making literature in medicine and other related disciplines.

This book is a distinctive and important contribution to this growing field. It combines a comprehensive critical analysis of a wide range of relevant philosophical, statistical, psychological and medical literature with an interesting set of experimental observations of primary care physicians. Dr. Ridderikhoff shows great erudition and wide command of a large reference literature. Dr. Ridderikhoff takes a firmly descriptive rather than prescriptive viewpoint on understanding clinical decision-making.

The key issues addressed in the book are 'How scientific is clinical medicine as a discipline?' and 'Do primary care physicians use inductive or deductive reasoning in their clinical practice?' In recent years following the seminal work of elstein *et al.* (1978) the emphasis in clinical decision-making studies has been on the hypothetico-deductive processes as the principal method of clinical reasoning. By contrast Dr. Ridderikhoff's experimental findings lend support to his assertion that induction is the method of choice for primary care physicians. This book has as it main strength (1) its form and realistic grasp of the philosophical foundations of clinical practice and (2) its perspective of the working clinician both in its critical analysis of the literature and in the design of the studies. Dr. Ridderikhoff has been influenced in his perspective by his many years in private practice before entering academic.

The book consists essentially of two parts. In the first part after a broad introduction touching on the philosophical and scientific complexities of the clinical method he focuses not only on utility and probability theories but devotes considerable space to a critical analysis of the literature on human thinking and problem-solving and on the nature of medical knowledge. He

tackles these complex areas with a clinician's eye but also with a firm foundation in philosophical analysis. The description of the Bayesian viewpoint is
highly critical with very effective use of the original texts especially those of
Von Neumann and Morgenstern.

In the second part of the book Dr. Ridderikhoff sets out to describe clinical
decision-making in primary care settings using simulated cases. He had one
major aim in these studies, namely, to try to establish by careful observation of
working clinicians in clinically realistic settings whether the predominant
method of clinical reasoning was, inducative or deductive. This was an ambitious agenda and the design and methodology are very explicitly described in
the book.

He has used a carefully selected set of cases which reflect the case-mix of
primary care physicians. The form of simulated methodology which he makes
use of reflects the wide range of possible questions and tests available to the
primary care physician. The studies were conducted in the physician's own
office and incorporated the time pressures found in real practice settings. The
verbal mode of interaction is used to reflect clinical reality. In order to be able
to decide whether induction or deduction is the method of choice he sets up
cognitive 'landmarks' in the experiments so as to be able to detect the key
differences reflected by the two methods under study.

The results of these studies strongly favour induction (in one or other of its
strategic forms) as the primary inferential approach used by primary care
physicians. Another important finding is that clinical experience seems to have
no influence on any of the measures of performance which he has developed
for this study!

This is a fascinating and provocative book which challenges our assumptions
about clinical reasoning. It will be of particular value to working clinicians,
teachers of clinical medicine as well as cognitive and educational psychologists
with an interest in medical education.

Thomas R. Taylor
University of Washington, 1988

Introduction

Do patients benefit from their doctor's advice? Do physicians know what they are doing? How do we know what the best advice is? Are the methods doctors use in medicine the most appropriate, valid, reliable, and efficient ones? Do our methods reach the standards of present-day conceptions of science? Or do we have to admit that medicine, as is often claimed, is an art, not a science? Must we allude to Kuhn's opinion that medicine is a craft, like calendering and metallurgy, or do we have to share Braithwaite's opinion that medicine is a science because of its 'natural domain'?

If we concede the former viewpoint then we are unable to answer the first questions. Art, in contrast with science, is based on experience, which is subjective, incapable of precise analysis, irreproducible, and impossible to measure. So we are facing the old problem of demarcation between the empirical sciences (theories, hypotheses, explanatious) and metaphysical concepts (art, prescience, pseudoscience).

But when medicine is not accepted as a science how can physicians possibly trace what they are doing? How can they trace the quality of their problem-solving, their decision-making? It will cast us in a dilemma as many people prefer the more personal approach of an art-like practice to the (assumed) more impersonal scientific approach.

We take the standpoint that in the interest of patients, physicians, as well as health care provisions, we have to make an effort to clarify the question of science versus art.

As is often the case with these big questions, a conclusive answer in the sense of a binary statement cannot be given. We can try to highlight a number of elements and features of both cultural domains. We can try to specify a number of characteristics of science as opposed to art. However, a clear definition, a world-wide consensus about 'science' cannot be found. So we have to take a personal standpoint in order to deal with the 'big question'.

According to my philosophical guide, Popper (1959, 1983), the aim of science is to find satisfactory explanations of whatever strikes us as being in need of explanation. A satisfactory explanation can be found in a theory which allows for genuine prediction. Whenever a prediction falls short of explanation from a theory, the theory has to be refuted. A theory or a conjecture belongs to the empirical sciences if and only if it is falsifiable. In other words, the theory must be able to specify under what conditions the theory can be falsified.

Verification cannot be part of the scientific reasoning as verification is some act of assuming regularities in nature upon which everybody relies in practice, but cannot be accepted as a valid inference (Hume, 1711–1776). Hume tried to show that any intuitive inference, any reasoning from singular and observable cases (and their repeated occurrence) to anything like regularities or laws must be invalid. But is this not exactly what doctors do in daily practice: reasoning from singular cases to general statements about the condition of the patient? Must we assume this way of reasoning as being scientific or as pseudo-science, or art? Can we infer from such medical statements valid explanations or predictions? Can we find some answers to questions like effectiveness and efficiency of the health care? These questions require a thorough understanding of clinical cognition and clinical reasoning. As medicine is predominantly a discipline which lives by its practical applications we shall first have to turn to the actual doings of physicians and face questions like:
– how do physicians solve problems?
– how do physicians make their decisions?
– do they employ special methods or strategies in order to reach a solution or decision?
– are these methods related to the structure of the medical knowledge?
– can this structure be specified in terms of a logical schema of statements and of classes of statements?

Methods in medicine

Raising the question about clinical strategies carries with it the assumption that there are specified methods used by the physician to solve patients' problems or to solve clinical research problems. Hardly anybody argues their existence but their specification is a matter of debate. Some people believe that there are strategies but that they are purely idiosyncratic: 'Each clinician has his own pathway to diagnosis' (Leaper et al., 1973). Others are convinced that physicians use one universal methodology in medical problem-solving (Elstein et al., 1978; Gerritsma and Smal, 1982). But Janis and Mann (1977) assert that 'people cannot be expected to use the same strategy for all types of decisions'.

Most people believe the doctor to use scientific reasoning strategies, or at least he should use these methods. However, a very large number of physicians disagree with this viewpoint as in their opinion, it does not meet the reality of the very personal approach to unique patient cases. Again it is the old question whether medicine is an art or a science (Forstrom, 1977; Munson, 1981).

Many theories in medicine seem to be scientific. However, over periods of time many beautiful theories, viewed as very scientific in their time, have been proven to be not within the scientific standard. The theory of excessive acid production in peptic ulcer was followed by the psychosomatic theory with a likewise change in therapy (v.d. Werf, 1985). Both theories had and have their ardent followers, who strongly believe in their 'scientific' basis. The 'local infection' theory for rheumatic diseases was believed to be a strong and scientific basis for causes and therapy of this disease. However, a couple of decades later it was silently superseded by the new theory of autoimmunity. Most theories in medicine have an aureole of science but put to proof most theories in medicine fail, although they persisted and still persist. Trotter called this 'the mysterious viability of the false' (quoted in Pickering, 1979).

After Pickering we can define science as 'a method of acquiring exact knowledge by observation, experiment, and measurement, leading to the formulation of a hypothesis that will explain the relationship between the facts observed'; and, 'by a scientific explanation is meant a logical deductive ratio-nalistic mathematical theory on quantitative measurements.'

However, most physicians do not consider their practising as a method of exact knowledge, as a logical deductive and rationalistic inference procedure. They assert their task as an art, preferring the personal touch to some imper-sonal strategy. Obviously, between these conceptions of art-like-practising and the explanatory requirements of medical science some tension exists. In the eyes of these doctors the caring, intuitive approach to patients is preferred to the explanatory inference of the diseased state. Especially in these cases physicians rely on the knowledge they have acquired in practice; their experi-ence. Experience is the knowledge physicians are particularly proud of. They often point to their – huge – experience as the main source of their cognition. Popper presented a patient case to Adler. Although the case was quite unfa-miliar to the great Viennese psychiatrist, he easily explained in detail the inferiority complex of the boy. Popper asking Adler how he could be so sure, got the reply: 'Because of my endless experience.'

Although this answer is very much recognisable to many physicians, espe-cially the experienced ones, it does not lead to a solution because of our ignorance about the real nature of experience. When the physician's knowl-edge is – largely – based upon experience, then we can ask, with the Scottish philosopher Hume, 'how do we know that the cases we have not experienced resemble the ones we have?' How could Adler know for sure that the present-ed case resembled the ones he had met in practice? How can anybody predict from previous cases the succeeding one? How can we conclude from a certain experience anything else than its similarity with some previous cases?

Brehmer sees this problem as the old controversy between inductive and deductive reasoning. 'Inductive judgment cannot be justified in the way de-ductive judgment can be justified. The judgment may very well be true, and serve as a guide in action, but it cannot be shown to be true. The fact that it works says little about its truth; it just tells us that it works, and the explanation why it works may be very different from what we think it is' (Brehmer, 1980).

However, if experience and personal knowledge play such great a part in medical practice, what is its relationship with medical science? Is it possible that we have to acknowledge the existence of two types of medical knowledge: a personal knowledge as practised in clinics and a general medical knowledge represented by textbooks, papers, reports, and so on? But how can we know that the contents of textbooks represents the 'official' medical knowledge and not the reproduction of the personal knowledge of the authors? In other words, how scientific is medicine as a discipline? How reliable are the causal explanations in medicine? For example, the coronary artery theory as explanatory for myocardial infarction has been proven to be untenable by the hundreds of cases with myocardial infarction without any traces of coronary vessel pathology. Still, the theory exists, apparently without any sign of reconsideration.

Theories in medicine are closely related to the conception of diseases as definable entities. When theories fail two possible explanations come forward. First, the causal relationship between the observed facts and the conception of the disease-entity remains unobserved or is wrongly interpreted. Secondly, the conception of the disease-entity is inaccurate, or at least dim. This notion refers to the core body of medical knowledge: the taxonomy of diseases. We shall discuss this matter at some length in Chapter I.

The misinterpretation of causal relationships can be attributed to inaccurate reasoning methods as well as the obscurity of these relations. The study of the reasoning methods is the fundamental part of this book. It is our conjecture that reasoning methods are closely related to the other part of medical science: the conception of disease and the mutual relationship between diseases and disease-classes. Viewing clinical cognition and clinical knowledge in their mutual relationship can be revealing for a number of suppositions about medical science. It may give rise to questions like, 'Can scientific methods be applied when the fundamental knowledge base is unscientific?' and, 'How can the input and the output of a medical decision process be valued when the contents of these items cannot logically be deduced?'

It is my impression that thus far the relationship between methodology and the nature of the related discipline has been neglected as a focus of attention. Thus far, much emphasis has been placed on the strategy or strategies that people, including physicians, ought to use. 'Instead we should concentrate on what people actually do and develop descriptive models to account for decision processes. This, then, has been the trend of late: from normative to descriptive modelling' (Howell, 1982).

For these reasons I decided on an investigation using a descriptive model of medical methods.

Planning and investigation

Lasegue, the famous French clinician, stated: 'Doctors observe little and they observe badly.' Being a doctor myself, apparently little hope is left for observing the essentials and the characteristics of the medical problem-solving and decision-making process. Fortunately, several investigators from different disciplines preceded me in outlining the theoretical and – sometimes – practical aspects of the physician's decision-making methods. However, these models mainly represent a way of reasoning which seems to deviate from what can be observed in routine clinical practice. They are predominantly based on the physician's description of his working-pattern. We agree with Sober (1979) when he states that 'the clinician's description of his clinical diagnostics is no more than a rationalization. It is false to the facts of his own psychological processes.' The schemas of most investigators are based on some kind of deductive reasoning. We believe this viewpoint to be too one-sided. It does not take into account the notions of the physicians about their habits and routines; their notion of the art-like approach to clinical practice.

Any investigation that does not take into account the real situation in medical practice is likely to fail as explanatory of medical methods. Or, as Biörck (1977) stated: 'This type of investigation has to be done by people who know what doctoring means.' It has also to be adapted to the level of health care at which the doctor really makes his decisions. Or, as Taylor (1976) stated: 'It is, therefore, more promising to begin projects of this kind with an analysis of the decisions made by the physicians in the appropriate area of the health care system so that from the beginning the proposed system will fit as closely as possible to the needs of the existing system and to the physicians who will use it.'

Therefore, we adopted another way of reasoning as possibly being explanatory of a number of physicians' inference processes. We based this method on the counterpart of the deductive reasoning: the inductive method. We can frame, therefore, the purpose of the study into the fundamental (research) question: 'Do physicians predominantly use a deductive or an inductive type of clinical reasoning?'

According to our design two prerequisites have to be formulated:
(1) there are two ways of clinical reasoning;
(2) the study has to be of a descriptive nature.

In order to be explicit and objective the use of a model is a necessary tool for observing. A model acts as a theory which can define the landmarks and the criteria according to which observable phenomena can be traced and recognized. A model can act as an unbiased guide leading us through the often obscure and scarcely visible directions and routes in the physician's reasoning processes. We cannot observe without a particular thought in mind; we are not blank watchers. In order to prevent intuitive or wishful thinking we have to make clear what ideas we have in mind. Explicitness enables the tracing and retracing of the thinking processes of the experimenter as well as those of the physicians-participants. It should be a necessary condition in descriptive studies especially in those studies in which the (cognitive) processes are difficult to access.

The doctor has to make decisions in an uncertain problem situation which involves two systems: his own and that of the patient. From this the main problem arises, because studying the functioning of the physician means observing these two systems which at the same time influence each other in a special implicit way. It is like focusing on a certain point on a turning wheel while sitting on another wheel rotating in an opposite direction. One observes flashes only partly recognisable.

The design of the model is a result of reflection and analysis from literature; literature from various disciplines like philosophy, cognitive psychology, informatics, medicine, and history. Within this design I needed both – philosophical – lines of reasoning in order to observe the doctor as solving problems and making decisions.

The second prerequisite refers to the clinical environment. The descriptive nature of the study implicates a scenario and a method of recording which enables the physician to operate in a way as natural as possible. It includes observation and recording in his own familiar office, interviewing the 'patient' in a verbal mode, free-questioning in every direction, adequate 'patient answering', customary time-limits, avoiding normative judgements, etc. Briefly, it was necessary to set the participant at ease, with the expectation of proceeding in his customary way. We must realize that some stress would remain as a normal feature of all medical problem-solving.

These prerequisites lead us to the following selection of problems to be overcome in the investigation:

(a) the – theoretical – modelling of the clinical reasoning methods;
(b) the highlighting of the landmarks within these methods in order to recognize and to observe their various behaviours;
(c) the choosing of a way of observation which enabled the testee to behave as naturally as possible;
(d) the elimination of mutual influencing of physician and patient by standardizing the 'patient'.

ad (a)

The theoretical conception for the modelling of the reasoning methods stems from the basic methods of scientific reasoning: inductive and deductive. Both strategies have their roots in ancient Greek philosophy. Their advantages and disadvantages have been a source of long and heated discussions throughout the centuries. Both camps have their adherents, their proponents and their opponents. For more than several centuries the English speaking world has been dominated by the opinion that scientific reasoning is of a special kind, inductive. This opinion has been so strongly advocated by such skillful and persuasive thinkers that even when many of the principles of induction have been repudiated or allowed to fade away we still remain in an unconscious bondage to a number of inductive practices and habits of thought. The influence of, for example, the philosophers Bacon and Mill, extends to the present day in which the great majority of investigators, at least in the medical world, follow the line of inductive reasoning, consciously or unconsciously. The method of induction is so interwoven with the traditional thinking in medicine, that most scientists are not in fact conscious of acting out a particular method. 'Most scientists are completely indifferent to – even contemptuous of – scientific methodology. However, the fact that scientists do not consciously practise a formal methodology is poor evidence that no such methodology exists' (Medawar, 1969).

The opposite direction, the reasoning from the general to the particular, the deductive strategy, is advocated as the method of choice in scientific reasoning. But advocating does not include practising. Deductive strategy includes the hierarchical ordering of hypotheses and knowledge base, as we can find in disciplines like physics and mathematics. The question is whether medicine can be treated in this way. Is the content of medicine structured in a way that it can compete with deductive reasoning?

Medawar proposed a strategy that occupied a position halfway between the above methods and called it – misleadingly – hypothetico-deductive. This method has been extensively described for the province of medical problem-solving by Elstein *et al.* (1978). However, on scrutinizing this strategy we must fall in with Harre (1972) declaring this strategy basically inductive. As we shall argue in Chapter II the same argumentation fits for the method of probabilistic reasoning. Probability theory can be seen as a supplement to inductive reasoning as it basically sets limits to our reasonable belief in an inductive statement.

So we based our modelling on these two types of reasoning: inductive and deductive.

ad (b)

The definition of the landmarks enables us to observe and to conceptualize the behaviour of each of the methods. As mentioned above, deductive reasoning comprises a hierarchical ordering of the hypotheses which are derived from the facts which cover the contents of the hypotheses (or theory). Between hypotheses and evidence exists a causal deterministic relationship. It means that the hypothesis h is completely compatible or incompatible with the evidence e; h is a full deterministic cause of e (Popper, 1968). The landmarks of deductive reasoning are a consequence of these basic features, as there are: the progression down the (hierarchy of) hypotheses-levels with increasing sharpness of the circumscription of disease entities; the consistency between hypotheses and evidence; and the refutability of the hypotheses.

Inductive theory insists on the primacy of facts: the classification of facts, the recognition of their sequence and relative significance. To these facts something is added which empowers the scientists to pass from statements expressing particular facts to general statements. Inductivism is mainly preoccupied with the justification and ascertainment of the evidence in relation to the discovery of a thought, a hypothesis. It typifies inductivism as a method in which the discovery (a hypothesis) and the justification form an integral part of thought. That which leads us to form an opinion is also that which justifies our holding the opinion (Medawar, 1969). Characteristics for the inductive strategy are the early hypothesis generation (comprising more than the evidence so far acquired) and its circular reasoning. The circularity of the reasoning arises from the mixing of what has to be explained (explicandum) and the conclusive or justifying explanation (explicans). In the inductive method the explicandum is justified by the explicans from which it arise. It means a reasoning from hypothesis to hypothesis via justification towards the next hypothesis, in which the intellectual processes are themselves the grounds for verification, and the evidence gathered for the justification procedure acts as new input for the generation of the next hypothesis. The landmarks follow from these characteristics including also the irrefutability of most hypotheses and the physician's choice behaviour.

ad (c/d)

'If you want to find out anything from the professional workers about the methods they use, I advise you to stick as closely to one principle: don't listen to their words, fix your attention on their deeds' (Einstein).

The doctor has to make decisions in a situation which involves two systems: his own and that of the patient. In order to investigate the problem-solving process, one has to freeze one of the systems. Studying the doctor automatically includes a 'fixed' patient. A 'fixed' patient is a simulated patient: a device which could serve as a patient, with or without the help of an intermediary. For our purpose of storing a large number of data, these data must be highly flexibly stored (and retrievable), have to cover a broad area of symptoms and signs, and should be easy to manage. In addition, the requirements of realism must be satisfied. We shall elaborate these thoughts in Chapter V.

The various types of patient scenarios should cover a large part of the clinical disease classes. They have to deal with a wide range of complaints, illnesses, physical, mental, and social dysfunctions.

A new simulation model was created on the basis of symptom configuration and classification. The symptom is defined as 'every functionally objective or subjective phenomenon which can be observed directly or indirectly and which is indicative of either an illness or condition of the patient.' The symptoms are arranged under 6 headings (another three headings are reserved for treatment and therapeutic management), while each symptom is accompanied by a more or less fixed set of aspects specifying the pecularities of a particular symptom. This configuration leads to a system with approximately 7000 entries which enabled the storage of information from 9 real life patients each representing a specific disease in different organ systems.

The sphere of reality was underlined by the use of the verbal mode for the physician-patient' interview. The mediator, a young physician representing the patient, could easily meet the demands of reality with regard to speed of answering and answerability. The videotaping of the scenario did not really disturb the sphere of 'normal practising'.

Medical science

Norbert Wiener, founder of cybernetics, referred to medicine as a semi-exact science and this is probably if anything a generous comment. Nevertheless, modern medicine is generally perceived as quite successful compared with the discipline practised, for instance, a hundred years ago. Epidemics swept the world, people died at a young age from tuberculosis, pneumonia, diphteria, etc. In those hundred years total life span rose from the mid-forties to the seventies, perinatal mortality declined 10–20 fold. So, in the light of these accomplishments, medicine must be a science, as science stands for progress, innovation and solidity.

However, few people realize that most of these victories can only partly be attributed to medical science. The discovery of bacteria cannot be ascribed to medicine. The cow-pox vaccination by scarification was introduced by the wife of the then English ambassador to Turkey. The proponent of the vitamin theory was a Dutch physiologist, the founder of chemotherapy a German scientist, the discoverer of X-rays a physicist. The extension of total life-span must be largely attributed to better housing, the construction of waterworks and sewerage, better nutrition, and an overall increasing welfare for the majority of the population. Great progress is made by the development of potent drugs to combat life-threatening diseases. Most of this development is effected by pharmaceutical industries. The fabulous technical improvements which have been incorporated into clinical practice and nursing give medicine an air of scientific basis and solid understanding, of possessing the truth. It conveys the impression that physicians and medical personnel know what they are talking about. It breeds the idea that health and illness are universally definable conditions; that, provided that intelligent reasoning is applied, the truth, that is the deduction and the solution to my diseased state, can easily be extracted from the symptoms and signs as presented by me.

It is exactly here, as is the case in many sciences, that differences of opinions appear. It must be an alarming thought that in the space of thousands of years medical science has not reached generally accepted definitions about the most fundamental elements in medicine like health, disease, symptoms and signs. More than a century ago the physician Oesterlen (1852) formulated a number of recommendations such as: 'to show, clearly and impressively, the mode in which we must proceed in our observations, investigations, and conclusions, in order that our theorem and problem may become more clearly intelligible, and that we may arrive at experimental truths and definite laws in our department of science, as well as at scientific principles in practice.' 'Still we have no concept of disease' (Sadegh-Zadeh, 1980); or 'What is disease? The absence of health. What is health? The absence of disease!' (Boorse, 1977). Tremendous differences exist between medical criteria used by the examining physicians and the relativistic socio-cultural standards employed by lay people to identify (the presence of) illness. More alarming, however, are the differences of nomenclature among physicians. Croft and Machol (1974) observed a 'lack of standard medical definitions' and recommended to study and to reexamine the entire taxonomy of diseases.

This book is not intended to boast of the achievements of medicine. It will contribute to the philosophy about the fundamentals of medicine, to a better understanding of its contents, and the way in which the reasoning faculties of practitioners can contribute to a generalised, cross-cultural, cross-situational discipline; in short: medical science.

Organization of this book

As a consequence of our starting-point we shall first discuss the fundamental issues, i.e., the contents of medical knowledge and its reasoning processes, as these two parts establish the heart of a scientific discipline. We take the standpoint that medical knowledge has two faces: one which can be defined as the generalizable, scientific face, the other the countenance of a medical knowledge as it is practised by medical practitioners all over the world. Therefore, it is essential to know what is really going on in the physician's mind. Chapters III and IV will be dedicated to typically human processes like: thinking, problem-solving and decision-making. These issues form the core body of the physician's work, in the offices, in the clinics, at family homes, on streets, ships and wherever doctors are busy.

The study of the literature on these matters leads us to the conclusion that little is known about the actual work of doctors. Little is investigated, nothing is definite, most of the hypotheses were based on belief or more or less superficial observation.

Being a medical doctor myself, with 15 years experience in family practice, I have several advantages in exploring physicians' behaviour in daily practice. I can understand what they are doing; I can understand the medical jargon; I have easy entry to their practices; ethical issues shall hardly arise; I can count on the co-operation of many of my colleagues. Moreover, I can handle medical data myself, I am more capable of creating an atmosphere of reality and trust during any investigation; I can converse and discuss the problems of daily practice, the inconveniences, and the responsibilities one usually meets in clinical practice. I can rely on a reasonable knowledge of medical literature; I can sense the inconsistencies and the gaps in disease descriptions; I can gather the medical data of the patients myself; and my experience enabled me to brush aside all statements typically inconsistent with the routine work of a (family) doctor.

I gained the confidence of some 30% of all family physicians in the city of Rotterdam. They, and some general internists, enabled me to perform this investigation into problem-solving and decision-making processes in clinical practice.

Chapters V and VI will be dedicated to the theories, the methods and the results of this investigation.

The conclusions of the study, and, more important, the consequences of the results, not only of the investigation but of the critiques on the pertinent literature as well, will bring the book to a conclusion in Chapter VII.

Where I succeed in bridging the gap between the reader and the often mystical world of medicine, and may encourage other investigators to a profound (re)search into this domain, this study will surely have attained its goal.

CHAPTER I

Medical knowledge

> In another two hundred and fifty years present
> day doctors may seem to our descendants as
> barbarous as Fagan and his colleagues seem to
> us. In those days, terrifying in black robes and
> bonnets, they bled the patients; now, terrifying
> in white robes and masks, they pump blood into
> him.
>
> (Nancy Mitford)

Introduction

Medicine is born of care for sick and disabled people. When in Mesolithicum the professional practitioner entered the scene the best he could offer was care and prayers. In the process of becominga scientific discipline medicine has always vascillated between care and cure, between the personal human touch and the strict application of modern techniques, between art and science. This background might explain the lack of generally accepted terminology and nomenclature. In more than 10,000 years medicine has not been able to provide a clearcut statement about the concept of disease, and can say even less about the concept of health. Every doctor carries his own concept of disease and, therefore, his own conception of the medical process which is the process which takes place between the entering of the patient into the health care system and his leaving. Symptoms and signs are personally appreciated and interpreted according to personal standards and norms. The aggregated symptoms lead to diagnoses meaningful only to the particular doctor who arrived at them. This can hardly lead to overall acceptable and unambiguous disease-definitions and a consistent and universal taxonomy of diseases.

However, when the doctor, lacking a clear taxonomy, cannot establish disease-entities, how can he forecast for the patient the natural course of the disease? Because by grouping the same diagnoses into a particular class we can learn to know what the process of that particular disease will be. Because it is the prognosis, the course of the disease, that counts for the patient and the doctor. Without the establishment of a disease-entity how can the doctor know which symptoms and signs are pertinent to the disease-entity? How can he determine the accuracy and precision of his data? How can he determine any treatment when he is unaware of the course of the disease?

Medicine is kept in a quandary between its art-like processes and its striving for scientific standards. It is our opinion, that medicine has not reached the standard of a universal and explanatory discipline.

A historical view

From the very start mankind must have suffered from diseases. Their existence was demonstrated by symptoms and signs indicating life-threatening situations, or at least some discomfort. These symptoms and signs were originally assigned mainly to metaphysical causes and formed certainly no part of a system, except of a superstituous system. In the Mesolithicum when the human race generally opted for a fixed dwelling place and started agriculture, the physician entered the scene. He was, as a consequence of mankind's habitual causal thinking, closely connected to religion or, in most cases, was part of it. Although some systematization was undertaken by the Egyptians, the first real ordering and organization has to be attributed to the schools of medicine of ancient Greece (Hellas). Especially the schools of the isles of Cos and Cnidos, facing each other in the Aegian sea, had their particular impact on the conception of medicine. As Boinet (1911) said about the rival schools, they stand for 'les deux grandes idées doctrinales qui reviennent sans cesse à travers les siècles apres de long détours et avec des fortunes diverses'.[1]

In the Coan writings we find discussion of the organism, the suffering, the illness, and the disease; in the Cnidian scriptures the description of organs, diseases, and disease-classification is predominant. The dispute between the two viewpoints lingers on to the present day. Physicians still argue whether medicine must focus on the unique case of the patient's illness or must restrict its task to the scientific approach of the adequate diagnosing of pre-established (taxonomic) disease-entities and their pertinent treatment.

This distinction can often be found to exist in the discussion between extramural and intramural medicine, between the advocates of primary health care and clinical health care. It is, in our opinion, the distinction between care and cure albeit the distinction seems to be rather artificial.

Galen in the second century (A.D.) tried to compromise between the rival schools by placing the differences in perspective and pointing out 'that, in the greatest number of cases, cleavage of opinion comes from the failure to distinguish between the particular and the general, such being the source of disagreement between physicians in respect to the use of barley-water, and between philosophers concerning the virtues of the soul'. However, Galen's efforts were never given a proper response. During the Renaissance the vehement discussions lead to two camps, the Hippocratians and the Galenians.

The schism between the two Greek schools was less one of doctrine than of method. That is to say, it was one between diagnosis in terms of experience, and diagnosis in terms of reasoning. Again, it is the philosophical difference which separated Cos from Cnidos more than the medical ideas. It is the difference between appreciation of the sick state of the patient and understanding the sickness.

As medicine in those days had less to offer by way of cure, the caring and

---

[1] The two great doctrines which returned incessantly during the centuries with varying success.

Hippocratic aspect of medicine was more prevalent. It took another 1400 years, in descent from the Platonic-Galenic philosophy, before attempts were made to construct a more organised body of medical knowledge as opposed to the less organised body of Hippocratist physicians. In France Guillaume de Baillou (1538–1616) and in England Thomas Sydenham (1624–1689) started new incentives to (re)organise medical knowledge in a Cnidian sense. Their efforts were most successful.

The next two centuries presented a picture of an enormous accumulation of observed disease entities, mostly named after their reporter. These were the centuries of a kind of Baconian 'Medical Novum Organum'. It was the ambition of learned men to attain to encyclopedic knowledge, to spread themselves over the whole realm of it, and laboriously to gather all its products into a Corpus or System (Allbutt, 1896). However, as the depth and extent of the observable facts seem infinite in all dimensions, the task must be inexhaustable.

It took another genius like Virchow to bring order and organisation into the nearly chaotic collection of diseases, illnesses, syndromes, aggregates, etc. He, and others, were only partially successful.

To the Hippocratians it became clear that a system uniform in its proportions and parts is impossible; or that, so far as possible, such a system would indicate not progress, but arrest of development – in a word, a stereotype. Although minor reorganisations took place, the general picture has not really changed since.

During the latter decades of the last century the physicial sciences entered onto the medical scene, which provided medicine with tremendous possibilities for basic research and the application of modern technology. It gave medicine its scientific countenance of high preformance and nearly unlimited possibilities. But fundamentally nothing has changed since Virchow. Diseases remain mysterious entities super-imposed with personal and socio-cultural flavours, taxonomies are felt to be inadequate for accurate classification, treatments are more often than not based more on personal appreciation than on logical reasoning, while the concept of health seems to be undefinable.

However, medical science has to insist on the generality of terms and concepts. Efforts to organise medical knowledge into a general applicable system were and are still undertaken. In the present day the introduction of disciplines like informatics and decision-making again urge medicine to make up its mind and press physicians to define clearly and uniformly their concepts and nomenclature.

At the outset of our study we met questions like: What is health? and What is disease? It is particularly in these questions that the two grand ideas of medicine present themselves as different doctrines. It prevents a general and unequivocal statement supported by all physicians in the world. Both opposing schools have their own conceptions and their own adherents. The Hippocratic philosophy is based on the notion of an individual unbalance of physical and mental functioning, while the Galenic conception arises from the notion of disease-entities fitting into an overall explanatory arrangement based upon degrees of affinity. It creates the distinction between the man who describes a case and he who writes about a disease.

Most doctors claim to diagnose in terms of experience, which relates the presented complaints to the personal and socio-cultural conceptions of the doctor. Crookshank (1926) wonders whether this reasoning leads to insight in diseases and to sound decision-making. He states: 'Always striving towards the simplicity of synthesis, they do not separate disease from the man, or man from his environment. Hence their study of epidemics as illnesses of communities, their therapeutic utilisation of airs, waters, and places, and their insistence upon personal effort, while causation is to them in each case an infinitely complex relation almost insusceptible of generalisation. Per contra, nature, to the natural diagnostician[2], may become less a subject of observation than an object of superstition, while distrust of classifications may beget mental untidiness; and the study of symptoms, clinical indecision and a neglect of origins, **if not an expectancy that slips into fatalism.**'

The schism between the two schools still exists, the dispute continues. Regrettably, the weapons are not arguments but dogmas and beliefs.

The concept of disease

'We in medicine are always arguing the question whether "there is" such a thing as disease and what "the nature of disease" is, while we have no concept of disease which can form the intersubjectively controllable basis for such a debate; chaotic ontologies hamper rational discussion and argumentation because everyone has his own explicit idea of disease; yet we do not hesitate to classify this or that phenomenon as a disease, or this or that person as diseased; the boundaries between medicine and other socio-cultural areas remain quite unclear; hence the blind respect that the layman has for medicine is easily abused to permit the uncritical extension of medical interpretations of events to all aspects of human life. We daily arrive at countless diagnoses in numerous social fields, not only in the hospital or in medical practice, but also at the requests of courts, employers, insurance companies, school authorities, etc.; we thus affect the lives of countless people and set far-reaching social processes in motion, and yet we lack a clear concept of diagnosis; nor does there exist any explicitly formulated diagnostic method which can suggest to us how individual physicians reach their supposed diagnoses and what they understand "diagnoses" to mean. We daily generate countless prognoses and etiological statements which underlie our therapeutic decisions, and yet we lack an understanding of "prognosis" and "etiology". The same holds for treatment itself because no standard of efficiency is available for its evaluation. In short, medicine is in danger of becoming a supervisor of society and the controller of human culture, although its foundations are extremely defective. As a consequence of these unfortunate deficiencies we have 20–60% or more misdiagnoses (Wagner et al. 1978, Wagner 1964), which certainly lead to at least as

---

[2] The Hippocratic one.

many mistakes in therapy and to malpractice. The responsibility for these failures is usually ascribed to the practitioner. He or she is reproached for not applying "the latest medical knowledge", and it is said that keeping up to the minute would have helped. This is an all too primitive view for at least two reasons. First, one cannot reasonably require that specialized, complex knowledge must be applied in order to reach a particular goal if one does not state at the same time exactly what the goal is and how the method of application is supposed to work. Such a demand is based, secondly, on the misconception that clinical practice is nothing other than the application of medical knowledge. Third, who can assure us that the "latest medical knowledge" is best? For in acquiring the "latest" knowledge central notions like "disease", "diagnosis", "prognosis", "etiology", and "efficiency" must again be relied upon, and these notions, as stated above, have an obscure meaning'. (Sadegh-Zadeh, 1980).

Sadegh-Zadeh expresses his utmost concern about medicine as it stands. It must be an alarming thought that during thousands of years medicine has not reached generally accepted definitions about the most fundamental elements in medicine.

The amazing fact is that everybody knows when he or she is ill, as well as any mother intuitively knows her child is ill. Malfunctioning, 'feeling unwell', pain, objectively or subjectively observable signs, etc. they all constitute a situation in which the human being recognizes himself as being ill. However, it is up to the doctor to categorize this state of 'un-health' as a disease. As Meehl (1977) says: 'The difference between illness and disease is what the patient feels when he goes to the doctor and what he feels on the way home from the doctor's office'.

The patient relates his state to several parameters in his environment: the observability of his lesions, the approval of family, of fellow workers, of friends; incapacitated functioning, and so on. These parameters are typically connected to social expectations, division of labour, the ideology and ulterior goals of given societies, current conceptions about disease, environmental conditions, and so on. The patient's idea of disease therefore reflects social and cultural standards of a given society more than a generally accepted and standard conception of disease.

Mechanic (1978) tells about a study of skin disorder (dyschromatic spirochetosis) in a South American tribe in which the disease was so prevalent 'that Indians who did not have (it) were regarded as abnormal and were even excluded from marriage'.

To the patient disease is a socio-cultural concept which may change in time as well as in ideology. There seems to be two different conceptions about disease: that of 'the patients', the laymen, the general population, and that of the doctor, the so-called professional opinion. The dyschromatic spirochetosis apparently was a disease to the doctor, and a superb state of health to the population. Doctors also attend to people who evidently are not diseased, like 'patients' for cosmetic surgery, or for contraceptive prescription, or attend to childbirth, etc. We cannot persist in the notion that all that doctors do or treat are ipso facto disease related. If that were the case the only healthy person would be the one who escaped medical attention.

On the other hand, there are diseases unnoticed by the patient. It has been said that pathologists doing autopsies in cases of sudden death often find it a mystery why the victim was not dead years before.

In the medical world both conceptions, that of the laymen and the 'official' one, seem to co-exist, but nobody can tell us when the physician is talking about the one concept or the other. We hypothesize that the 'laymen's conception' correlates with the equilibrium idea of the Hippocratian school. This thought is a tempting one as de-stabilisation will clearly be noticed by the patient whether it concerns minor oscillations or more unbalanced conditions. This thought is perfectly reconcilable with the 'unique case' conception of the Coan school. In this conception the patient is his own yardstick with regard to the degree of unbalance, the deviation from his own 'normality'. It excludes the notion of normality being some kind of intuitive statistical normality. The notion of 'statistical normality' typically belongs to the formal conception of disease-entities. It presupposes the existence of some medical system such as the Cnidian school sought for.

The 'equilibrium' idea does not exclude the notion of recurrent configurations of similar or comparable patterns. But these patterns do not act as a means to a disease classification but as a basis for typology: as the classification of diseased people. This thought rejects the Linnean idea of systematisation by means of a fixed classification of observed patterns. As Allbutt (1896) states: 'All attempts to describe diseases in terms equivalent to the genera, species, or natural varieties of plants or animals are, then, erroneous; they lead to mistakes both of theory and of practice, and to ignorance of the underlying unity in the various forms of a disease. A sick plant or animal is but itself in another state, a state more transient and less useful.'

In 'Prognostics' Hippocrates begs the reader not to regret the omission of the name of any particular disease, since it is by study of symptoms in each case rather than from accounts of named diseases that the desired knowledge is aquired. Terminology and nomenclature are not essential features in the Hippocratic conception; names are but 'provisional formulae which, if permitted to harden into aphorisms, become fetters of thought' (Allbutt).

In contrast the Cnidian's aim was not an assay of the patient's state but the identification of his malady with a predefined entity. To this end the defined entities have to be part of a system that divides and subdivides diseases into a finite number of varieties or species. This classification becomes an expression of affinities, and takes a larger meaning and a conceptional summary of permanent and universal convenience. In this conception diseases are more or less stable entities, identifiable and classifiable into a universally accepted system of diseases. Within this framework nomenclature and terminology must be unambiguous and standard.

Scadding (1972) set forth the requisites for a formal definition of disease:

(1) avoidance of tautologies;
(2) definition of relevant populations;

(3) establishment of normal standards;
(4) universal acceptance of terminology;
(5) confidence in establishing the presence of each disease;
(6) flexibility to allow for modifying the definition due to changes in diseases with time.

The Galenic conception allows for distinction between diseases regardless of the individuals. It was assumed that a classification system, like the botany classification of Linne, could contribute to exactness and to accomodate physicians in unambiguously diagnosing diseases. Diseases could be classified as objects or groups of objects in nature: in Sydenham's words ' to be reduc'd to certain and determinate kinds, with the same exactness as we see it done by botanic writers in their treatises of plants' and possessing 'certain distinguishing signs which Nature has particularly fixed to every species' (quoted in Crookshank, 1926).

It is the thought that the adequate defining of diseases would enable us to group entities of uniform design into a reference class. The accumulation of uniform elements into a predefined class would enable us to recognize, to deduce, to learn about the particular element in order to present a valid judgement.

The fashion of classification restarted mainly in the 18th century and has given rise to the discipline of nosology or the taxonomy of diseases. Although this discipline has a strong impact on the medical image and the conception of disease and health, we believe the Hippocratic view still to have a strong and dominant foothold in present day medical thinking.

Taxonomy of diseases

'The process of classification, the recognition of similarity and the grouping of organisms and objects dates back to primitive man. He must be able to perceive similarities in stimuli for survival. The study of classification has always had two major interrelated components: 'how do we classify?' and 'how should we classify?'. The first component belongs to the domain of the psychology and philosophy of sense perception: What is similarity?, how do we know we recognize similarity?, how do we perceive regularity and relationships?, what are the criteria?, how does classification affect everyday life?, etc. The second component is the subject matter of taxonomy, the science of classification'. (The theoretical background of classification is borrowed from Sokal, 1974.) From these components three characteristics have to be distinguished:

(1) there must be something to perceive, to identify;
(2) we must be able to place these identified objects into a class of similar objects; and
(3) we have to know how these classes are to be interrelated.

Identification will be defined as the allocation or assignment of additional unidentified objects to the correct class, once such classes have been established by prior classification. The definition of classification is the ordering or arrangement of objects into groups or sets on the basis of their relationships. Finally, the definition of taxonomy will be defined as the theoretical study of classification including its basis, principles, procedures and rules. We can exemplify this with an example taken from botany: take, e.g., a flower. One could easily identify it as being cultivated or not, but it needed a genius like Linne to set up a taxonomy of plants in order to provide the possibility of finding the exact class and subclasses and name. Finally, a more or less experienced person must be able to find the category and name of the plant.

All classifications aim to achieve economy of memory. The world is full of single cases. By grouping numerous individual objects into a class, a taxon, the description of the taxon subsumes the individual description of the objects contained within it. By grouping the plant into a taxon we are already aware that, although not all the plants may yet have been grouped there, eventually all the flowers of the plant (these plants) within the taxon will be e.g., yellow.

Another purpose of classification is manageability. The objects are arranged in systems (which may or may not be hierarchic) in which the several taxa can be easily named and related to one another, e.g., the Mendeleiev system for chemical elements. The paramount purpose of classification is to describe the structure and relationships of the constituent objects to one another and to similar objects and to simplify these relationships in such a way that general statements can be made about classes of objects.

It is easy to perceive structure when it is obvious and discontinuous. But much of what we observe in nature changes continuously in one or another characteristic.

Classification that describes relationships among objects in nature should generate hypotheses. In fact, the principal scientific justification for establishing classifications is that they are heuristic and that they lead to the stating of a hypothesis that can be tested. (Heuristic is meant here as a force stimulating interest as a means of further investigation.)

Two kinds of classification can be distinguished.

(a) Monothetic: classes differ by at least one property which is uniform among the members of the class;

(b) Polythetic: the group or sets of individuals or objects share a large proportion of their properties but do not necessarily agree in any one property. No single property is required for the definition of a given group nor will any combination of characteristics necessarily define it.

Medical classification obviously falls within the latter distinction. In the polythetic classification there is a strong need to weigh characters, especially those that highlight the class to which they belong. But how to weigh? Should certain characters be weighted more heavily than others? Who determines the relative importance of the characters to be weighed? It is important to note that most classificatory labour is not based on fundamental scientific principles but largely on considerations of practicality. This practicality often leads researchers to weight discordant characters less than others.

The difficulty with such weightings is that one needs an initial classification to provide weights for the characters. But once classifications are established there is a reluctance to change, especially when the classification is assumed to be correct (Sokal, 1974).

In medicine a firm basis for classification was laid by pioneers like Morgagni and Virchow, using gross morbid anatomy and microscopy to explain the clinical manifestation of a great number of diseases. From the second half of the 18th century onwards the diagnostic process was directed towards the name of a disease, explaining all or many of the phenomena observed. Regrettably, the history of medicine almost always deals with 'ideal types' which are approximated, for the majority of disease-entities, and ultimately defined explicitly by their joint pathology and etiology.

In medicine, the classification must take into account both the history of disease in nature and the history of disease in persons, both universal and singular phenomena. Therefore, the capacity to form a unifying theory is severely restricted (Gutman Rosenkranz, 1976).

Difficulties arise because of poor definitions. But they also arise from an ill-defined classification, descending from the morbid anatomy classification of the pathologists of the last century. The physician observes, inferes, deduces, induces, etc. what is presented to him as the patient's problem, and translates these observations into symptoms and signs, more or less causally related, to a proposed disease. The pathologist classifies what he sees. But what makes that which the pathologist observes classifiable as disease? Both the physician and the pathologist provide a basis for claiming that physicians observes symptoms and signs.

But this claim places an excessive authority on the observations and assessments made by the physicians. The large amount of literature on observer and assessment variation seems not too encouraging in this respect. The interpretation is left to the doctor. That means:

(1) a subjective interpretation of the observed symptoms and signs (when observed);

(2) a subjective judgement about the aggregated symptoms and signs ('diagnosis').

It might be obvious that the subjective judgement depends on the physician's disease conception. It makes a world of difference whether he is supporter of the Cnidian style or the Coan one. In the latter conception any judgement is a unique one. The disease is assumed to be a particular state of the individual whereas the other school stresses the similarity and recurrent presentation of particular symptom-groupings as predefined. Where the Cnidian doctor looks for constancy, the Coan doctor searches for perturbations, deviations from the normal balance of function.

Whereas the Cnidian doctor is interested in all symptoms and signs very similar to the 'ideal type' of the disease-entity in the nosologic system, the Coan doctor will look for characteristics that distinguish this patient from another. In the former case the similarity of a symptom-configuration to a predefined disease-entity will be proof of diagnosis, in the latter form the recognition of a particular type of patient is the prevalent goal.

It is especially here that confusion in terminology occurs. The Hippocratic doctors employ usually the nomenclature of the formal nosology, which they have learned in medical school. They use it in order to express themselves in what they assume is a common language. By doing so they mix the two conceptions which leads to confusion and poor communication among physicians. Without explicitly defining their concepts doctors are completely unintelligible among themselves.

Medicine is not a subject in which terminology and nomenclature (prerequisites for understanding and insight) find their best exemplification. The matters of our inquiry, not having relatively fixed specific characters, do not lend themselves as yet to the construction of an appropriate terminology. Without fixed and generally accepted nomenclature names of diseases become empty shells expressing nothing more than some sort of convenience. Or in the famous words from Goethe's Faust:

> 'Denn eben wo Begriffe fehlen, Da stellt ein Wort zur rechten Zeit sich ein'.[3]

No part of the Platonic writings is more useful than those Dialogues in which the disputant is forced to feel how imperfectly he understands the phrases in common use. It was reserved to Aristotle to recognise 'equivocal terms' as a class, and to assign to them a particular name.

Physicians communicate in abstract terms to give their ideas the air of generality. But as Bloor (1976) stated, 'In truth there is no such thing as one precise and definite signification annexed to any general name, they all signifying indifferently a great number of particular ideas. It is one thing to keep a name constantly to the same definition, and another to make it stand everywhere for the same idea; the one is necessary, the other useless and impracticable'.

The generality which a clinical assessment, say a diagnosis, is supposedly to contain is not in its name. The assessment is general insofar as it stands for all other particular ideas of the same sort for the same physician. The very lack of visibility of these differences may assist in their perpetuation.

Subjective observation and interpretation of symptoms and signs, incomplete knowledge of morbid processes, poor definitions, and different viewpoints create great impediments to the generation and/or completion of a generally accepted taxonomy of diseases. Classification by genesis can be the expression of the order of our thoughts; and it is by the study of the aberrant processes that we may often detect the more intimate kinships which may provide us with elucidating insight into the concept of diseases.

Some remarks on the subject of international classification of diseases would seem to be necessary. In spite of its name it has little to do with the kind of classification we have just discussed. I prefer to reserve the name Taxonomy for the latter form of classification. The international classification refers to a statistical approach on diseases. Once a solid taxonomy of diseases (or nosology) is established it might be profitable to determine the size of the particular

---

[3] When meanings are lacking, a word will appear in time.

classes. At least it provides us with strong foundations for health care policy, ideas about shifts of endemic or epidemic diseases, the amount of health care personnel required, etc. It might also be a source for research and the gaining of insight into disease behaviour, e.g., from predictions based on large numbers.

The need for such a classification (of diseases) was first formulated in 1893 by the International Statistical Institute. It originated an International List of Causes of Death, I.C.D. This classification was revised every decade. The sixth revision of 1948 enlarged its usefulness for morbidity applications by increasing the specificity of rubrics and by emphasizing manifestations of disease rather than etiology. For family medicine a related system (ICHPPC) was developed by the W.O.N.C.A. (World Organization of National Colleges, Academies and Academic Associations of General Practitioners/Family Physicians), and is now under the aegis of the World Health Organization. In the light of the above discussion on the taxonomy of diseases it should be clear that any assessment based on the categories of ICD or ICHPPC should be judged with much scepticism.

Medical data

I

On becoming a medical datum

Patients entering the physician's consulting room present neither symptoms nor data. Symptoms are a medical translation of a patient's feelings where data are artificial elements preferably written in a (alpha)-numerical way based upon the symptoms of the patient. But even before a certain feeling of a patient can be acknowledged as a symptom or a datum a number of conditions have to be fulfilled. (We shall disregard the very complicated question of data related to the patient's social and environmental background. The processing of these data does not belong to the classical corpus of knowledge of the physician; this information is predominantly processed intuitively guided by experience.)

(1) *The 'sick role'*
Before the individual is acknowledged as a patient (the 'sick role', Parsons, 1951), his feelings must be acknowledged as belonging to a possible disease or disability. This depends on:
  (a) disruption of normal functioning;
  (b) visibility to others;
  (c) perceived seriousness;
  (d) evoked embarassment;
  (e) expectation of effective treatment;
  (f) incapacitating symptoms;
       and so on.
This makes it very hard for a physician to cope with the patient's problem. Tremendous differences (see, e.g., Mechanic, 1978; Friedson, 1970; Scheff,

1963) exist between medical criteria used by examining physicians and the relativistic socio-cultural standards employed by lay people to identify (the presence of) illness. Patients entering the 'sick role' have their own thoughts about disease. Because the 'sick role' provides a person with certain privileges, this thought is not free from personal values. The doctor's role is to define illness, confer the sick status on potential patients, establish priorities, and take the initiative in evaluating health status and controlling health problems (Brody, 1980).

(2) *The complaints must convey a medical significance*
When the presented complaint cannot be related to a – known – disease-entity or some disturbed state of health, it is generally ignored by the physician. There are two possibilities for denying the symptom:
   (a)   the complaint indeed cannot related to any known disease entity, e.g., 'Doctor, when I blink my right eye, I feel an itch in the little toe of my left foot';
   (b)   the physician is unaware of the existence of the disease to which the symptom can be related. This possibility arises when the disease in question is – extremely – rare (globally or in his environment), or there really is a gap in his knowledge memory.
To elaborate this further there are a number of communications about particular features in physicians' behaviour, like:
   –   he only considers the prominent symptoms as he has know them from past illnesses (Adlassnig, 1980);
   –   the physician is too prone to see things in patterns (Balla, 1980);
   –   he only looks for positive answers. The power of the positive response is more than 100 times greater than a negative one for a single attribute (Blois, 1983);
   –   during physical examination, a sign is noted when certain sensory stimuli have been recognized by the doctor. Errors can occur before the stimuli reach the doctor's mind because of sensory defects. Alternatively the doctor's cerebration may still fail to recognize and identify the entities (Feinstein, 1973);
   –   most physicians take into account the unreliability of patient's answers, physical signs, laboratory tests, reports, etc. (Dornfest, 1981).
When we consider the pace at which the physician conducts his practice, the inevitable overload of information and the extreme variability of problems he deals with (especially for family physicians), we can appreciate the extreme difficulty of both data collection and the generation of a reliable data base in clinical practice.

(3) *Degree of deviancy*
The symptoms and signs presented by a patient must be significantly different from the normal range before they are acknowledged as such by the physician (Feinstein, 1973). Problems may arise in deciding that such data is in fact different because of:

(a) a lack of reference values for most symptoms and signs in medicine. Of course, everybody has some intuitive perception of norms, but such norms vary in relating to socio-cultural values and current conceptions of medicine. Different physicians place different emphasis and interpretation on deviations from the normal in similar clinical situations (Anderson *et al.*, 1976). Striking differences in interpretation are found between physicians when performing estimations of, e.g., the attributes: 'obesity', 'thinness', or 'normal weight' (Lahaye *et al.*, 1978);

(b) the difference of presentation of complaints and bodily signs by the patient. Zola (1963) described the different types of presentation of complaints by Italian versus Irish patients and their physicians' reactions. Mechanic (1972) has also described the social psychological factors affecting the presentation of bodily complaints.

Reliability of data

Although the reliability of a symptom, the precision of the questioning procedure and the accuracy of the truth of the patient's complaint, cannot be assessed in numerical terms (Wulff, 1976), the carefulness of the medical procedure is often considered as a qualitative norm. The relevance of the symptom is often seen in its relation to a particular disease. The diagnostic value of a symptom is disease-conscious and its relevance is likely to be different for different diseases (Cumberbatch and Heaps, 1976). In the probabilistic version of the Galenic conception this relevance is often expressed as a weight accorded to each symptom for each disease. The disease which produces the largest ratio of the patient's weighted symptoms to the weighted sum of all characteristics for that disease is considered the correct diagnosis. As has been said, it presupposes a firm relation between symptom(s) and disease(s).

Regrettably, it is not as simple as that. Every physician knows that the same symptoms can have different meanings not only in regard to different diseases but to the same disease also. Pain in the breast with a younger man can be indicative of a pneumothorax, while in an elderly man it can point to a myocardial infarction. It can make a lot of difference if a symptom comes in an acute, an intermittent or an insidious way, even if it concerns one and the same disease.

Symptoms are the physician's interpretations of observable features presented by the patients and, therefore, subject to variation. Intra- and interdoctor variation have been widely recognized to exist. The variability may well account for the great differences and disagreements (i) between different physicians' data bases, and (ii) within one data base over time. The suggestion that feeding back clinical information to physicians so as to reduce the differences among them and improve the diagnostic performances is improbable (Lahaye *et al.*, 1978).

Information gathering is the accumulation of a profile of data concerning the patient. There are innumerable 'facts' to be gathered and there are many reasons why physicians can misinterpret data that they collect. This may be especially true for data with which the physician is less familiar, e.g., laboratory and X-ray results. Physicians often feel reassured by laboratory tests that they neither need nor really use. Zieve (1966) listed 10 items concerning misinterpretation and abuse of laboratory tests. The present 'habit' of ordering multiple tests does not contribute to a clearer understanding of the problem nor help with diagnosis. They are only helpful when:

(a) all test results related to a particular disease are normal thus tending to exclude a disease;

(b) all test results related to a disease are abnormal thus tending to confirm that disease.

They are least helpful when some are positive and others negative for the same disease (Griner *et al.*, 1981).

The interpretation of the result is also influenced by the definition of the cut-off point, the point where the calibration changes from normal to abnormal. When this point moves towards a disease specifity increases but sensitivity decreases, and as it is moved in the direction of non-disease, the reverse is true.

This problem in the interpretation of results contributes to observer error. It is the physician's job to observe. However, as we have discussed before, observation is said to be 'theory-laden': our attention is drawn to specific pieces of evidence in a situation because we have hypotheses which impute relevance to some of them and not to others (Popper, 1972). A purely neutral and indifferent collection of clinical facts is not possible.

Each observation is contingent on the person, time and place. What makes for real difficulties in constructing a reliable data base is that these value-laden data give rise to several errors in data processing storage and retrieval. These can be:

(1) errors of observation: neglect or failure to observe, poor interpretation;

(2) errors in recording: only a limited number of symptoms, perhaps only relevant to the doctor, is recorded. (see also Nobrega *et al.*, 1977);

(3) errors of memory recall: inaccurate recall of assumed similarity of patterns; inadequate retrieval (fail to find recorded symptoms, therapies, etc.);

(4) errors of classification: incorrect classifying of patients into the data system.

These errors give rise to a number of questions, like:

(a) what is the magnitude of observer error?

(b) how can this error be minimized?

(c) what is the significance of the residual variation? and

(d) what are the effects of observer variation (Gill *et al.*, 1973).

Two types of observer variation can be detected:

(I) the variability of observation and recording by one physician of repeated observations (intra-observer variation), and

(II) the disagreement of observation and recording between two or more physicians (inter-observer variation) of the same phenomenon.

In literature these features are described in two ways, dependent on viewpoint: intra/inter-observer errors and intra/inter-observer agreement.

The review of Koran (1975) discusses intra- and inter-observer agreement as observed in literature. Intra-observer agreement for a number of physical signs values ranged between approx. 60% and 80%. The inter-observer agreement scored lower, ranging from about 40% to around 80%. It was noticed that the more diagnostic categories there were to consider, and the less severe an abnormality, the lower the inter-observer agreement. From all sources of information history taking is the most important but also the least accurate. Agreement among physicians concerning the patient's history was only 2 in 25 patients (Stern *et al.*, 1975).

According to Gill *et al.* (1973) the error rate in diagnosis due to observer variation forms a small proportion of the total error rate in diagnosis. In fact, somewhat less than one quarter of all diagnostic error can be attributed to the acquisition of 'faulty' data by the doctor.

In order to be reliable medical data have to fulfil at least three requirements:
(1) stability, or reliability across time, for the same judge and the same data;
(2) consensus, or reliability across judges, for the same data and the same occasion;
(3) convergence, or reliability across the data sources, administered on the same occasion and interpreted by the same judges (Card, 1977).

The fulfilment of these requirements is most often wishful thinking. Natural variation and human interpretation makes medical data less reliable than one would wish. Moreover, inadequate registration of data, when observed, creates another obstacle to the creation of reliable data bases. A data base is an important tool in building the foundation of medicine or of the specialty it concerns. We physicians are urged to search and research for guidelines in delineating reliable medical records and medical data bases. However, Cochrane *et al.* (1951) comment: 'Although medical disagreement has long been recognized as common and was published by Alexander Pope (1723), there appears to be some general reluctance to recognize it as due to the subjectivity of medical judgment and even more reluctance to investigate it quantitatively'. And that is hardly a reassuring thought.

Data recording

Medical records are of the utmost importance to the medical practitioner and his patients, and, when legible, to his colleagues while attending to the practice. However, both Donebedian and Kroeger identified problems of completeness and accuracy of the medical record (Gardiner, 1979).

Data processing in medicine is a method by which the data base is transformed into a problem list. It is the important step whereby information gathered about the patient is filtered and the clues are selected and grouped into meaningful problems (Cutler, 1979). However, an ideal data base has never been formulated. The medical record is too often accepted without proper criticism (Goldfinger, 1973). Often physicians are blamed for their inappropriate records, but one has to admit that there are few guidelines for physicians. A major attempt to streamline the medical record has been published by Weed (1970). He stated that the Problem Oriented Medical Record (P.O.M.R.) can help in ameliorating a variety of difficulties now besetting medicine, among which are:

(1) medical problems dealt with or without context;
(2) inefficiency in practice;
(3) lack of continuity in care;
(4) the apparent inapplicability of 'basic science' facts and principles;
(5) inefficiency in education;
(6) the absence of meaningful audit in the practice of medicine;
(7) increasing complexity;
(8) explosion of technological tests;
(9) withdrawal or apathy of the supervisory personnel.

All these obstacles to good clinical practice are fully recognisable, but they cannot all be blamed on the medical record. We agree with Feinstein (1973) stating that 'the medical record was a reflection rather than a cause of the difficulties; a symptom of the intellectual maladies but not the disease.'

Weed's P.O.M.R. was an attempt to standardize the medical database. Unfortunately, this did not much alter the main problem with clinical data, namely, its reliability. While being the advocate for the P.O.M.R., Weed forgot to define what the problems are. The difference compared to the conventional recording was the remodelling of the source-structured recording into a problem-structured one. In so doing, he moved the record into a kind of vacuum, because people cannot handle problems as singular data, nor is there any explicit or implicit context in which to process them.

Data collection is inefficient when the information collected does not lead to the formulation of useful hypotheses or to the testing of existing ones and may, therefore, be circumstantial or irrelevant. Besides, data have to be assessed to determine whether the information is true. Next, the data have to be evaluated to determine whether they reflect an altered body state or are a normal variant (Young, 1982).

But all these sensible considerations do not alter the actual situation. Let us have a look at an actual situation, a physician-patient encounter. The patient, usually ill at ease, presents his or her complaints expecting the doctor to take serious notice. The doctor knows from experience that he must behave in a way that would at least not discourage the patient from telling his complete story. Continuously making scribblings certainly does not belong to this behaviour. The doctor asks some questions and sometimes notes down the patient's answers. But when answers cannot be related to the pertinent questions they become meaningless, unless the questions are standard, which they are commonly not. Evidently, the doctor should note down the answers as well as the pertinent questions. This would certainly involve him in great difficulties of extensive and time-consuming registration of data. But it would also bring him into conflict with the patient, who expects a serious conversation with a human being, not with a writing robot. The sensible physician takes the intermediate position: he records those items that seem important to him and to the case at hand. For all other data he uses abstract words; words he at one time learned from formal medical language. These abstract words contain sufficient information for him at that precise moment and for that particular patient. No more, no less.

It is certainly not what scientists consider to be optimal, but surely it is the way it is. And when the critical scientist comes to his doctor he certainly does not expect a writing robot.

Diagnosis

Medical diagnosis is a difficult and complex task largely empirically based and poorly understood as an intellectual task. The gap between the information which is present for diagnosis and the information accessible from memory is difficult to close even for a highly trained general practitioner with substantial daily exposure to many disorders (Eddy and Clanton, 1982).

There is no general agreement on the term 'diagnosis'. Originally the word means to 'distinguish'. In this sense, diagnosis can be viewed as the process of differentiating between a number of alternatives. This assumes that there actually are 'things to be chosen'. This preconception implies three more basic assumptions:

(a) in the Cnidian approach, the distinction between one disease-entity and another;

(b) in the Coan approach, the recognition (of the characteristics) of a particular type of diseased individual;

(c) the distinction between health and disease.

Generally speaking, the former two possibilities are the more common idea of the term diagnosis. Differentiating between existing diseases or diseased states is usually viewed as one of the physician's major tasks.

But the physician has not only to differentiate between disease alternatives, but between disease and health as well. Not every patient who enters the health care system is – medically speaking – ill, while not every diseased person is considered to be ill in social life. As we have previously described, health and disease are largely abstract concepts which can be based on time, social and cultural factors. The tension between these concepts makes diagnosing, especially in primary health care, very complex. Judgement about the patient's state of health or disease can raise conflicts between the patient's judgement about his well-being and that of the physician.

Current medical knowledge provides physicians with little help in making (objective) judgements about the question: 'ill versus not-ill'. Nevertheless, society expects physicians to decide these questions in matters of insurance, social security and employment. Definitions of both states are left conveniently vague. They certainly do not allow physicians to decide unambiguously between ill versus not-ill.

We can agree with Gross (1977) that only generally accepted definitions of the states of health or disease can provide support for the physician's judgements in, e.g., insurance and employment evaluations. However, these definitions and descriptions do not exist. There are tremendous differences between medical criteria used by the examining physicians and the relativistic sociocultural standards employed by lay people to identify the presence of illness. This does not mean that those diagnosed as 'not-ill' according to the medical criteria were not suffering from some measure of discomfort, unhappiness, or inefficiency because of their symptoms (Kellert, 1976). Brown found that non-sickness accounted for almost 25% of the diagnosis made on 12,835 patients: patients who labelled themselves as being ill. In England Balint estimated that 25%–50% of all patients who go to doctors are not suffering from any pathological entity or nosological syndrome (quoted in Drucker, 1974). Approx. 60%–70% of people who experience some discomfort do not go to an official medical institution (Mechanic, 1978).

The very notion of 'diagnosis' is rather vague, so that to deal with it in terms of algorithms may only give the discussion a superficial and spurious exactness. One author tells us that diagnosis is the prerequisite to accurate prognosis; a second, that diagnosis is the method of distinguishing between diseases that have symptoms more or less alike; and a third, that a correct and integral diagnosis is the *sine qua non* of rational therapeutics. It must be obvious that the art of 'diagnosis' reflects the views of the physicians with regard to their conception of a disease.

It is from one of the writings of Hippocrates that we derive the clearest notion of the Coan diagnosis whereby, after full examination of all relevant detail, related phenomena were simply interpreted in the light of past experience, the resultant judgement being expressed descriptively yet concisely without the confusing arising from the hypostatision of abstracts and the pluri-interpretable use of names. Hippocrates says in the First Epidemics book that he framed his judgements or *diagnosed* by paying attention to what was common to every and particular to each case; to patient and prescriber, to general constitution and local mood, to habits of life and occupation of the patient; to his speech, conduct, silences, thoughts, sleep, wakefulness, and dreams; to his tears, stools, urine, spit and vomit; to earlier and later illnesses; to sweat, chill rigor, hiccup, breathing, belching, passage of wind, bleedings and piles.

From this Hippocrates diagnosed the patient according to the theory of the natural elements (e.g., melancholy = black gall) and the particulars of the patient which leads to the recognition of special 'types' of diseased people which enabled him to foretell the future course of the diseased state.

Quite contrary is the Galenian way of diagnosing. In the New Sydenham Society's Lexicon 'diagnosis' is described as the 'distinguishing of things, the noting of symptoms whereby a disease or plant or *other* object may be known for what (it) is and not another'. In the same fashion Hélian published his 'Dictionnaire du Diagnostic, ou l'art de connaître les maladies et de les distinguer exactement les unes des autres'. It is a deterministic approximation such as we can also find in recent definitions. For instance, 'The diagnostic process employed by a physician can be seen as an attempt to establish the similarity of the presenting symptoms and signs of the patient to a particular disease prototype' (Gorry, 1974).

In this vision diagnosis is the recognition of a set of symptoms representing a prototypical disease-entity. The set of symptoms does not necessarily have to be complete. As Allbutt remarked, diagnosis depends not upon all facts, but on crucial facts. However, by virtue of a lack of clearly defined disease-entities, we are unable to determine which symptom is crucial and which not. Moreover, it is expected that the symptom-disease relationship can be a probabilistic one. According to Card (1970) there is a calculable chance that a particular symptom (indicant) is related to the prototypical disease-entity. This probabilistic version of the Galenian way of diagnosis is especially elaborated in the discipline of clinical decision-analysis. In this discipline the diagnostic process is considered to be a sequential process in which the physician employs a test to obtain more (probabilistic) information in order to test the new information, and so on until a 'final hypothesis' or 'diagnosis' is reached. Every step in the process is considered to be quantifiable by means of numerical (probabilistic) values.

This conception presupposes a number of prerequisites:
(1)   a clear and unambiguous concept of disease;
(2)   a standard taxonomy of diseases;
(3)   a rather fixed group of symptoms representing a disease;
(4)   that doctors diagnose according to a process of sequential steps.

With regard to the first three conditions we have already discussed the obstacles and impediments related to any kind of medical standardization. In Chapters 2 and 5 we shall pay attention to the last condition.

The probabilistic version of the Galenic way of diagnosis is a new version of an old theme. Its application (which is merely in the context of rational clinical decision-making) is limited by lack of definitions and standard terminology. Not the method but medical knowledge itself hampers the employment of all those formal decision-making models which have been created during the past thirty years. Medicine has not made up its mind about its most fundamental element: disease.

In the diagnostic act the different viewpoints about the concept of disease are reflected; and as we shall argue later on, the same is true for the diagnostic method. In essence, medicine still faces the dilemma of its inadequate definition of its basic feature, the basis upon which medicine itself is founded.

Prediction

'Doctor, what is going to happen with me?' is the essential question which the patient addresses to his physician. He may ask it in somewhat different ways but the essence remains. He is not really interested in the name of the disease except to distinguishing between catastrophic (e.g., cancer, heart disease) and non-catastrophic (e.g., influenza, superficial infection) diseases. Besides, medicine has invented, and still invents, lists of – especially to patients –

meaningless names, or adjectives like rheumatic, essential, idiosyncratic, etc., which really mean nothing. The patient is also not interested in the names of the medical treatment apart from some global indications such as drugs, operation or physiotherapy. The physician has been provided with an innumerable variety of drugs under fancy names, differing from country to country, covering only a couple of thousand chemical compounds. The patient, and who is not, is interested in what lies immediately ahead of him. Unfortunately, making predictions is very difficult. The same applied to the physician, although it is often assumed otherwise. He has the advantage over the layman that he has some knowledge about the natural history of the disease just diagnosed in the patient. Supposing the diagnosis and the classification to be correct, the physician has the knowledge or can find in the textbooks some general statements about the course of the disease.

However, textbooks are usually very silent ou prognosis. Most textbooks refer to three possible outcomes: favourable, unfavourable, and dubious. To say that this is a meagre assessment of outcomes is an understatement. Prognosis should be the ultimate, the paramount goal of medicine. The Linnean System for botany laid the foundations for major advances in agriculture. It enabled agricultural scientists to predict with high accuracy the outcomes of certain crops or species. It provided the basis for scientific investigations like those of Mendel, de Vries, Morgan, etc. It laid the foundations for modern genetics, one of the topics in modern biotechnology. In a similar way the classical taxonomy of chemical elements enables chemists not only to deduce but also to predict the qualities and characteristics of newly developed chemical compounds.

The lack of a high quality taxonomy of diseases and the absence of well-founded predictions, therefore, may not be coincidental. Without a well-founded prognosis based on a well-founded diagnosis how can we be sure that the actions taken in the interest of the patient will give a favourable result? Without a well-founded prognosis how can the doctor be sure what he is doing? His aim is and must be the alteration of the course of a disease in a favourable direction. But when we are unaware of this course how can we possibly decide upon any action (including non-action) that will lead to the desired goal?

In general, three types of actions can be distinguished:
(1) in the case of a self-limiting disease, no action has to be undertaken to change the course;
(2) the disease has a more serious character, and therapy is – easily – available: the physician will not hesitate to influence the course;
(3) the disease is fatal, no causal therapeutic action is really known.

The physician will try and prescribe all kinds of actions known to mitigate and alleviate the symptoms and possible incapacitating outcome of the disease. It presumes a triad of conditions:
(a) the diagnosis is correct;
(b) the natural course of the disease is known;
(c) the actions and effects of the proposed therapeutic management are known.

The first condition has already been discussed in detail. About the second condition the natural history of most diseases is unknown. What we do know about the natural history of diseases is derived from medical knowledge from the past fifty to a hundred years. Nowadays, practically every patient is 'treated' with all the means medicine can provide. We are therefore only able to observe a therapy-modified course of a disease, superimposed by varying reactions to the therapy.

This leads us to the problem of the third condition: when we introduce some therapy, e.g., a particular drug, into a patient, whose diseased state has an unknown course, how can we possibly know what the (re)actions of this drug are? Without the possibility of making accurate predictions how can we possibly know that we shall reach what we want to reach? Or in the famous words of Mager: 'If you don't know where to go, you may very well end up somewhere else, and not even know it'.

The most fundamental characteristic of any medical action is its selective nature; doing one thing precludes doing another. It is selective in two ways: selective as to the nature of the therapy, and selective as to who receives the therapy. One can only study the reactions of one drug in one patient, excluding other and/or similar drugs. And our actions are selective as to the receiver in that while giving some kind of therapy it precludes the not-giving of it. When we direct our attention to those who receive the therapy other problems are posed. What are the selection criteria for the particular drug? Is the physician especially interested in this disease? Which patients with the disease will be selected: the most ill ones or less ill ones, men or women, old or young, etc. Or is the physician especially interested in the drug itself? When the physician chooses the most ill patients he will almost inevitably find a change in their condition. Where the patient improves, there may be a very likely alternative explanation to this finding: because of his higher or lower judgements between the first and the second encounter he observes simply a regression effect.

Turning our attention now to the validity of the judgements, it is necessary to disentangle the effects of the treatment. This can only be done by random distribution. But this is not likely to happen since the resources are usually scarce and the randomized sample is not always randomly distributed. Action is always selective, meaning that as we select certain cases for treatment, we by that very act also select other cases not to get treatment. The only cases we can observe, therefore, are the true positives and the false positives. Subjects tend to focus only on the number of true positives, i.e., they follow the strategy of using only confirming evidence (Brehmer, 1980).

Prediction is medicine's almost exclusive and powerful instrument for measuring the effects of treatments and the performance of physicians. With regard to the former, the necessity to establish criteria with regard to the results of treatment becomes more and more urgent. In the time of Alexander Fleming things were easy. Physicians and the whole medical world had a clearcut notion of the natural histories of the known infectious diseases. The introduction of penicillin gave clear results in the cases of certain infectious diseases. Nowadays, we can only rely for most diseases on rather sketchy descriptions of courses of diseases, maybe obsolete. To deduce anything from the predictions of these diseases seems rather optimistic.

Without proper and accurate prognosis it becomes extremely difficult, both for medicine and pharmacy, to develop and, moreover, to test new drugs and therapies in order to judge them as a substantial addition and improvement to the pharmaceutical and medical arsenal.

Treatment

Treatment should be the easiest part in the whole medical process, from data acquisition to prediction. Once the course of the diagnosed disease is outlined the choice among a group of well-organized remedies should be seen only as dotting the last. But, as elsewhere, confusion is the rule. Non-specificity of remedies is common, chemical compounds waiting for a disease, yes, even treatments for non-diseases, are all part of this confusing picture. Most antibiotics and antirheumatics are non-specific, antihypertensive drugs are applied for the prevention of some kind of vascular disease which may or may not occur; doctors treat healthy people with cholesterol-reducing drugs although there is no proof whatsoever that cholesterol plays any role in provoking a disease.

Nevertheless, when one takes a glance at the contents of most medical journals, the number of papers about all kinds of treatments is impressive. Some journals are exclusively dedicated to – mostly – drug therapy. One may wonder why so much attention is paid to a subject that is, as I argued before, of no great importance to the medical process. Drugs and therapies come and go, the latest hardly any better than the previous (ones).

Of course, it is essential to keep in touch with developments in the medical and pharmaceutical world. But real innovations in pharmaceutics are rare. After the discovery of penicillin in the late 'thirties, the principle of antibiotics has not changed. The first benzodiazepines were introduced in mental health care in the beginning of the 'sixties, and afterwards hardly anything has changed with respect to the basic compound, except for an overwhelming variety of derivations, all with similar qualities to the basic substance. Many drugs have existed for decades without any change. Of course, one can point to the (small) number of fields of success. The substitute therapies like hormone and vitamin therapy have gained great success. The antimicrobial drugs have greatly improved the prognoses of patients with infectious diseases. Advanced surgery has saved many lives. But the fields of success are restricted. For most of the common ailments adequate solutions are not available. One need for the abundance of articles, reviews, surveys, books, etc., on treatment. Nevertheless, medical congresses are predominantly dedicated to therapy. Sessions for physicians are almost exclusively dominated by one subject: treatment. So there must be an explanation for this remarkable phenomenon in the medical world. We can think of two possible explanations.

(1) Often, and especially in primary care, the physician is confronted with an unclassifiable complex of complaints. No diagnosis or only a rudimentary

one can be made, while the patient is in trouble, or supposed to be. The patient looks expectingly at the doctor, whose lack of relevant medical knowledge leaves him empty-handed. The only thing which remains is to act like the ancient Greek doctors and prescribe drugs for the various symptoms, without possibly knowing what the (re)actions will be. Every communication with a colleague in a similar, or assumed similar, situation is to be welcomed. Every hint in literature, even the remotest, may be of help in forthcoming acute or chronic but unexplained cases. For diseases for which a cure is unavailable or unknown, various types of drugs are prescribed. Feinstein (1967) states: 'every treatment is an experiment', but we have to realize that it is not a scientific experiment. The drug is seen as a tool in the hands of the doctor; an extraordinarily powerful tool without which no health can be gained, no real help can be offered. 'Are you quite sure, doctor, that there is no other drug for my complaints?' Instead of issuing a resolute denial, the physician prescribes another drug of which he has vaguely heard. He is part of the belief in health and of the health bringing medicaments as they are loudly advocated in the news media.

(2) The physician makes a straightforward diagnosis. He can choose among many widely available and powerful drugs. Within a couple of days the patient will be cured or at least restored from the most incapacitating symptoms. But where the illness persists or even deterioriates, there may be a number of possibilities:
(a) it is a variant of the natural history of the disease;
(b) the disease, or cause of the disease, is resistant to the drug;
(c) the patient is not compliant with the advised regimen: e.g., he does not takes the tablets as prescribed;
(d) the physician made an inaccurate diagnosis.
It is approximately in this order that the physician considers these alternatives. Although the latter alternative may be the most probable one, it often does not enter into the physician's consideration, because the physician's personal judgement and commitment about this case (and diagnosis) hamper an objective and renewed view.

Every physician is acquainted with a great number of variants. Needless to say, these variants, if existing, are unmentioned in the textbooks. Every physician feels a need to compare his variant and its treatment with those of colleagues, verbally or through the literature.

Resistance to particular drugs is often mentioned in a somewhat vague and general way (it has to be distinguished from specific items like the resistance of a particular bacteria to a specific antibiotic). It is often blamed for a number of disturbances like: insufficient resorption, insensibility to the drug, pharmacological processes, etc. In these cases a similar drug is prescribed, with varying results. To be in touch with all possibilities of 'resistance' the physician consults other experts and experienced colleagues, and of course various sources of information.

Literature about non-compliance is growing. The importance of this problem is unknown. Although this issue can be viewed from various viewpoints the term indicates that it is the patient who is to blame for his infamy in not following the physician's orders. 'And the doctor knows what is good for you'. A number of alternative explanations can be thought of. Some of them will be discussed in Chapter III.

Unmentioned, thus far, is acting in an emergency. Sometimes the physician has to initiate a treatment before a diagnosis is made and approved. Fortunately, these emergency cases are relatively rare in practice and do not require an extensive knowledge of pharmaceutical compounds. In relevant cases only a small number of drugs is used. Janis and Mann (1977) listed some conditions to this emergency decision-making:

(1) awareness of serious risks if no protective action is taken;
(2) awareness of serious risks if any of the salient protective actions is taken;
(3) moderately high degree of hope that a search for information and advice will lead to a better solution;
(4) belief that there is sufficient time to search.

Most doctors are very much aware of the serious risks. As students they were taught about alarming symptoms in terrifying diseases and the frightening consequences to the patients and to themselves in case of misjudgement or inadequate action. Every medical student remembers lectures in which the teacher presented a patient case in which he, the teacher, saved the life of the patient in a heroic action at the last moment. And every student made a mental note to act swiftly and heroically if he were ever to be confronted with a similar case, or an assumed similar one.

As the number of protective actions is relatively very limited the risk in undertaking such actions is rather small. The doctor's main concern is the panicky reactions of relatives and neighbours of the patient. In case of nose-bleeding, as I was told as a student, the first thing a doctor has to do is to get rid of the family! It is amazing how much time then is left for consideration and search for rational solutions.

Each physician has to be aware of his actions. Powerful drugs, extensive surgery and other interventions make the consequences in contemporary medicine so far-reaching, that no one can afford to stay in the wings.

Summary

In this Chapter we discussed medical knowledge from the viewpoint that there may be two sides to the coin, the concept of disease. We sketched a side dominated by the personal appreciation and interpretation of the symptoms and signs as presented by the patient. This Hippocratic view takes into account all facts of the patient whether it is his medical history and physical signs, his medical and social background, or his environmental situation. It leads, and must lead, to a very individualised judgement about the condition of the patient. The judgement is, in the words of Sadegh-Zadeh (1981), 'a particular statement about an individual and relative to the patient to whom it applies; it is relative to the physician, his conception of disease, his medical knowledge, and time.'

The other side of the coin is the scientific side, that side of the formal taxonomy of diseases and clearly defined disease-enitities. This side is assumed to be universal, well-established, standardized, and declarative. The conception of disease is anchored in and adjusted by the taxonomy, unrelated to physicians' opinions. The disease concept is one of a strictly definable pathological entity constituted by (groups of) symptoms and signs in causal patho(physio)logical relationship bearing in it a clear notion of prediction. In this view the process of diagnosis is merely 'a distinctive characterisation in precise terms'.

Both sides of the coin bear their positive and negative consequences. When we assume the concept of a disease to be a personally appreciated condition of disturbed health then we run into an ambiguity concerning the medical data. The patient's information must convey a certain medical significance or else it will remain unobserved. But if it is a personal concept the quality of the medical significance can only be attributed to the doctor's opinion. That would give medical data an individualistic and particular flavour, and be, at the same time, largely uncomparable. It can account for the differences in medical assessment which may arise from differences between doctors in their particular ideas about disease-entities, symptoms, and signs. These differences must be attributed to the personal appreciation of the case at hand and some contempt for explicit and uniform names. Judgement, in the Hippocratic way, relies heavily on experience and personal knowledge. It is hardly explicit and can only be communicated by example. As Hippocratic physicians largely use the nomenclature of the 'scientific' side of the coin, matters are greatly complicated.

On the other hand, the 'scientific' version very much lacks a consistency of contents. A well-defined and well-founded taxonomy of diseases is as yet not established. The current taxonomy is certainly not universal and declarative; it lacks consistency and a firm structure of internal relationships. An explanatory classification of diseases must rest upon an analysis of all patho(physio)logical processes which would enable us to trace the more intimate processes of diseases, beginning with those of the widest generality and moving onwards to the more specific. However, in general, this explanatory classification is still in its infancy. This specifically applies to the domain of primary health care with its early stage symptom-configurations.

As a result of an inadequate taxonomy and subsequent terminology the reliability of medical data cannot be determined. In the absence of clear definitions of diseases the validity and reliability of clinical data, generally speaking, can only be appreciated as personal interpretations, as degrees of belief. This ascertainment implies an impediment to the construction of reliable clinical databases which may act as a source for decision-making and clinical research.

Neither the Hippocratic nor the Galenic diagnosis have that firm consistency which guides to a reliable prediction. The prognosis, as the ultimate goal in the medical process, can only be deduced with any certainty when we learn to know the average course of a particular disease. But in that case we shall have to define clearly the disease in question, determine the correct reference class in the taxonomy of diseases, diagnose as clearly as possible this specific disease, and start investigation with regard to the course of this particular disease.

The differences between what should be and what really happens are most clear at this level. Generally, apart from personal experiences, we have only a slight notion of the prognosis. As these experiences can hardly contribute as reliable evidence to the body of knowledge, a reliable judgement about treatment still awaits. Treatment should be guided by the course of the disease; treatment should push the course of the disease in a favourable direction. But when the desired direction is unknown, any statement about the quality of the treatment must be given with great restraint.

It must be clear that to make any statement about diseases, diagnoses, symptoms and signs the investigator has to provide and present the medical data in a standardized and uniform way. Diagnoses must be specified in their particular configuration of aggregated elements. Only by pursuing these strict rules can the processes and their outcomes be made comparable and be classified.

Chapter II

Ways of reasoning

The use of hypotheses is the method of science. To suppose we can make discoveries by the Baconian method is a delusion. A hypothesis or supposition is not a conclusion; it is only a starting point for methodological observation and experiment, the endeavour being not only to prove it, but to disprove it.

Hughlings Jackson

Introduction

The aim of science is to find satisfactory explanations of whatever strikes us as being in need of explanation. The aim of our study was (and remains) to discover and to explain certain elements of physicians' behaviour in regard to problem-solving and decision-making processes. Our hypothesis has been that physicians use special methods in problem-solving. More specifically, we guessed that these methods might possibly be the methods used in scientific reasoning. Medical education brings students into contact with scientific methods. We assumed that this contact has a lasting influence and affects their rational behaviour in clinical practice.

However, the implications of this hypothesis were far-reaching because science appeared to be not that monolithic structure that most people, including myself, assumed. When science is defined as a way of reasoning which can guide us to the revealing Truth, several ways seem to lead to Rome. Of old two different ways have existed, each with its own camp of adherents and supporters. But, assuming that physicians use scientific methods in their daily practice, which one is employed? Which type of reasoning could be a model for their mental processes? We decided to model the two principle scientific methods: the deductive and the inductive. The characteristics of each model must bear comparison with the characteristics of the clinical processes as we have observed them among the physicians participating in this study.

To be declarative we first had to study these scientific ways of reasoning in order to model these methods and to discover their characteristics. The study not only revealed a number of characteristics but also the strengths and weaknesses of these methods. It brought to light the often thin line which lies between scientific truth and personal belief, between wisdom and expedience. In particular, the discussions and disputes between the two camps were very instructive for an understanding of the qualities of the methods.[1]

[1] See, e.g., Lakatos, I. (ed.): *Inductive Logic*, 1968.

In studying the methods it became clear that the inductive process is the more common one, the every day strategy. It is a method mainly based on experience and personal knowledge. It allows quick decision-making and fast action. It is the method of survival in a dangerous world. In contrast, the deductive stratagem is a more laborious and tiring method unsuitable for quick decisions, but superb for understanding and insight. The deductive stratagem is the more rational, 'scientific' way of reasoning while the inductive method allows for the human touch, the admission of emotions into the process.

Whether there is some form of inductive logic (a justification of the inductive method as a scientific method) is still a matter of fervent debate. The introduction of probability theory into inductive reasoning changed its status but lessened the validity of the conclusions. Induction misses the strength and force of the deductive process, but can act as an incentive to scientific research.

In the last section of this Chapter some fundamentals of the probability theory will be discussed. Although the discipline of mathematical statistics marshalled several weaknesses of the inductive process, the application of probability theory is hampered by its own strict conditions. These conditions, especially the rules of large numbers, are certainly a stumbling block in the case of medical investigations. In clinical practice large numbers and reliable estimations are hard to find.

An intermediate method, the hypothetico-deductive, has been proposed to solve some of the problems which are met in inductive reasoning. In our opinion, this alternative suffers many of the shortcomings that can be observed in inductive reasoning. We shall shortly comment on this method.

Science and belief

The use of scientific methods in medicine seems obvious, because the power of science is to make contact with reality in nature by recognizing what is rational in nature, i.e., the discovery of laws which will be generally applicable. We can regard as scientific any purposeful human activity designed to provide tentative and refutable hypotheses about the nature of events, which means, in clinical medicine, the name of a disease explanatory of a number of observations in the patient. Feinstein (1973) advocates a scientific approach to diagnostic reasoning. However, most patient-physician encounters seems to be of an implicit character. Physicians appear to dig into their bag of cognitive tricks, and use whatever strategy seems most appropriate in a particular situation at a given moment. This varied repertoire used in medical inference has not yet been decomposed or broken down into sets of formal procedures, nor has it been shown to be decomposable in such a manner (Blois, 1983). Because of this implicit character physicians are largely unable accurately to break down their diagnostic thought processes into explicit, understandable steps.

It seems that the whole process of diagnosing and confirmation ultimately relies on our own accrediting of our own vision of reality. The physician is merely drawing a portrait of his conceptually prefigured conclusions, while not knowing how he arrived at them. This is the usual process of unconscious trial and error by which we feel our way to success and may continue to improve on our success without specifically knowing how we do it, for we never meet the causes of our success as identifiable things which can be described in terms of classes of which such things are numbers.

Moreover, since every act of personal knowing appreciates the coherence of certain particulars, it implies also submission to certain standards of coherence. All personal knowing appraises what it knows by a standard set by itself (Polanyi, 1958). This implies that we credit ourselves with much wider cognitive powers than an objective conception of knowledge would allow, but at the same time reduces the independence of human judgement far below the extent traditionally claimed for the free excercise of reason.

We still continue to feel that there is some consistent relation between our beliefs and the factual evidence presented to us. We can regard this (with Hume) as a mere habit, without acknowledging any justification of the convictions expressed by this habit. Belief is the strong subjective feeling to which we have committed ourselves. Facing contrary facts means recommitting oneself; this is usually asking too much. In this sense there will always be some discrepancy between someone's belief and the truth. Bertrand Russell defines 'truth' cynically as a coincidence between one's subjective belief and the actual facts; and it is impossible to say how the two could ever coincide.

The answer to this dilemma is that what we view as actual facts are in reality accredited facts; accredited to our interpretations and personal views. Our observations are directed by what we think to see, or what we ought (to ourselves or to others) to observe. No one seriously believes that the mind is a blank slate upon which the senses inscribe their record of the world around us. We are directed not only by our personal knowledge and belief, but, by the mere fact of subjectivity, we are committed also to our statements. Reconsidering the statement means denying one's personal belief in it. We would never use a hypothesis which we believe to be false, nor a policy which we believe to be wrong. As Darwin stated: 'How odd it is that anyone should not see that all observation must be for or against some view if it is to be of any service'. Popper makes this point for his pupils: 'My experiment consists in asking you to observe, here and now. I hope you are all co-operating and observing! However, I fear that at least some of you, instead of observing, will feel a strong urge to ask: 'What do you want me to observe?' And, as Bacon stated, 'the last thing anyone would be likely to entertain is an unfamiliar thought'.

The subjectivity of our observations gives our beliefs the mark of universality, of truth, as we want it to be true. Any presumed contact with reality inevitably claims universality. The claim of universality opens possibilities for creating a system based on subjective beliefs. The remarkable stability of such a system is based on two factors. First, any contradiction between experience and a mystical notion is explained by the reference to other mystical notions. For instance, mutilation as part of the rites to enter adulthood, as are habitual in many tribes, is justified by the presumed protection against any disaster in the future; the truth of this prediction can never be verified or falsified.

Secondly, stability arises from the automatic expansion of the circle in which an interpretative system operates. For instance, in social systems the failure of regulations or laws is met by other regulations and laws with equally uncertain outcomes and consequences. In medicine the unproven theory of a causal relationship between myocardial infarction and coronary artery pathology is met by an equally unexplained theory of coronary artery spasms. No matter what comes up, there will always be some explanation ampliative to the current system.

This is cynically phrased by Asimov (1976): 'In fact, so eager are people to believe the essentially incredible that they will resent, even with violence, any effort to advance evidence in favor of disbelief. If some mystic, with a wide and ardent following, were to disown all his previous statements, if he were to declare his miracles frauds, and his beliefs charlatanry, he would lose scarcely a disciple, since one and all would say he had made his statement under compulsion, or under a sudden stroke of lunacy. The world will believe anything a mystic will say, however foolish, except an admission of fakery. They actively refuse to disbelief.' And the world is full of 'mystics' in social, political, administrative or religious spheres.

The assumed accuracy of observation automatically yields improved certainty of predictions. By predominantly implicit rules of inference we guide our practical knowledge and observations to a firm prediction. Every gambler uses his own implicit rules of inference to predict the highest gain, time after time, scarcely shocked by negative outcomes, time after time. The 'Intellectual Cripple' hypothesis of Slovic implies that humans may well be little more than masters of the art of self-deception.

The implicitness of the rules confers a sphere of authenticity to the actions of people. The physician's action is considered more authentic than what he says he is doing. Without explicit knowledge of the rules, the practitioner is more like a connoisseur. We trust in connoisseurship as we trust in artistic expertise: it cannot be questioned. Connoisseurship, for example, can be communicated only by example, not be precept. But submission to this kind of artistry would derive us from learning the rules of inference, and therefore the possibility to retrace our steps of reasoning. It should be science's prime concern to elicit these rules. But, as Medawar (1975) says, 'one cannot but wonder at the fact that scientists themselves are so seldom deeply interested in scientific methodology'.

It is assumed that in logic we can find the rules for the ideal form of reasoning. This form includes attempts to discover the rules for valid and sound arguments, rules which can direct our thought in the pursuit of truth. Our principle goal is to avoid drawing false conclusions from true evidence. A physician is always trying to avoid arriving at false diagnoses given reliable data from the patient. However, the active perceptive physician can always fall into various traps. For instance, the point where one starts in a process of reasoning will be those statements or principles which one supposes one knows, or for the moment pretends one knows in order to discover their consequences (Harre).

The truthfulness of the conclusion can only be based on the correctness of a number of predictions contained within the conclusion. However, as we discussed in Chapter I, prognosis is not an exemplification of validity and reliability in medicine. There are several traps which can lead the doctor to fallacious prediction. It requires a firm conception of explicit rules to elicit the medical reasoning process, or, as Popper says, 'in order to deduce predictions one needs laws and initial conditions: if no suitable laws are available or if the initial conditions cannot be ascertained, the scientific way of predicting breaks down'.

Methods in science

Like the dual views on the concept of disease, methods in science also have their duality. Both methods claim to be the correct way to the truth, both maintain their own set of inference rules. Both theories have their own camp of adherents, who are often entangled in long and fervent debates. When we ask 'science' to assist in eliciting inference rules as they are used by people like physicians, we shall, regrettably, have to face this dispute. 'Scientific reasoning' is not that universal and unique way of reasoning that is often assumed. Both methods have in common the idea that scientific discovery starts from speculative thought, but the inference, the method of reasoning towards an explanatory theory, differs greatly.

In the deductive scheme the conjecture, the bold statement, is severed into a hierarchically and logically bonded set of hypotheses in order to reach a specified hypothesis which can be verified or falsified (preferably falsified) by (simple) experimentation. In induction the speculative thought mainly arises from observation. The inference is directed at the claim of universality of the idea as it was induced from the observations made. Whereas the deductive method aims at a construction in which a single test can be a proof for the total hierarchy of hypotheses (and therefore the statement), the inductive method tries to collect verifying instances to support the theory.

This latter method is the so-called Baconian method, The scientific method starts from observation and experiment and then proceeds to theories. Bacon's method rested on induction by simple enumeration. Collecting all sorts of cold, warm and intermediate temperatured bodies and elements he hoped by listing all the qualities of these bodies and elements to find (induce) universal laws of nature with regard to heat.

The inductive method is assumed to be the more 'natural' type of scientific reasoning. We believe scientific progress to proceed by way of induction, i.e., the sudden flash of insight, the 'Eureka phenomenon'. We believe that Archimedes found his law by coincidence, that Euclid discovered the axioms overnight, and that Newton formulated the law of gravity after he was struck by a falling apple. But when these events occur, they occur very seldom. These thoughts normally do not spring into one's consciousness. Several pre-thoughts may have been slumbering all the time. At a sudden and most unexpected moment the ideas come together to form the illuminating hypothesis. The discovery of penicillin by Alexander Fleming did not occur as a sudden flash of insight (as is often believed) but was the end point of a long process of putting several observations and ideas into a combined hypothesis after years of hard labour. Relativity theory had a long history of preceding ideas but it required a genius like Einstein to entertain that one unfamiliar and illuminating thought that brought the preceding ideas together into the revolutionary hypothesis.

Contrary to the deductive hypothesis, the inductive statement stems from observation, commonly not from theories or ideas. It means that the inductive statement is related to our mental and emotional state. This certainly forms a threshold in formulating bold conjectures. As Bacon said: 'the last thing anyone would likely to entertain is an unfamiliar thought'. Several ideas, constructions, securities suddenly appear to be out of order. It affects one's feelings of certainties, of the laws of nature. Maybe these laws are less valid and reliable than they seem to us, but actually they generally form an integral part of one's subjective beliefs and commitments. The reflecting person is then caught in an insoluble conflict between a demand for an impersonality which would discredit all his commitment and an urge to make up his mind which drives him to recommit himself. Therefore, we shall rephrase the Baconian statement into: 'The last thing anyone would be likely to entertain is a state of uncertainty'.

Inductive reasoning, therefore, is a relatively safe way of reasoning. It does not go far from our views of reality and it verifies instead of falsifies a particular hypothesis. Inductive inference allows people to collect data pertinent to the statement. It is the picking up of data which can sustain one's preconceived idea. It also disregards data which can disprove and it does not lead people to (re)consider alternatives open to inspection.

To avoid prejudiced thoughts and, moreover, prejudiced conclusions, probability theory has been introduced in the inductive inference method. By sorting out coincidental from non-coincidental events, natural phenomena from biased observations, probability calculation can make distinctions between what might be real and what represents our prejudiced thoughts. However, the introduction of probability theory does not solve all the problems of the unwarranted inductive conclusions because of its own limitations. Probability hypotheses do not rule out anything observable; probability estimates cannot contradict, or be contradicted by, a basic statement; nor can they be contradicted by a conjunction of any finite number of basic statements; and accordingly not by any finite number of observations either. No matter how often we have seen white swans it does not lead to the conclusion that all swans must be white. We shall discuss this issue in more detail in the section on probabilistic reasoning.

As an alternative to the inductive method a third method has been proposed. By the middle of the nineteenth century it had emerged from philosophical scriptures (e.g., Whewell, Pierce) as an alternative to the induction method as advocated by Mill.[2] The scheme tries to combine the older methods

[2] John Stuart Mill, British economist and philosopher, 1806–1873.

by allowing one to start from an inductive statement but demanding the application of deductive inference rules as rules of logical statement transformation. 'Once we have formed an opinion we can expose it to criticism, usually by experimentation; this episode lies within and makes use of logic, for it is an empirical testing of the logical consequences of our beliefs' (Medawar, 1969). We shall shortly describe and comment on this method in one of the following sections.

We shall now describe and discuss at some length the various ways of reasoning.

Deductive reasoning

Deductive reasoning means: from theory to facts, in which the various steps take the form of a logical ordering (hierarchical nesting). It is usually stated in the form of a syllogism. For instance,

All Greeks are mortal (major premise)
Socrates is a Greek (minor premise)
_____
Socrates is mortal (conclusion)

As this syllogism is meant to be valid for all kinds of situations it can be transcribed as,

$$\forall_x (P_x - Q_x)$$
$$Pa$$
_____
$$\varphi_a$$

Or, for all persons in all situations (general premise) applies for this particular person (specified premise) this particular result (specified conclusion). It may be clear that the conclusion follows inescapably (logically) from the former premises and can be traced back. We shall exemplify this type of reasoning with an example from physics borrowed from Braithwaite (1968).

The system has one highest-level hypothesis:
  (I)   Every body near the earth freely falling towards the Earth falls with an acceleration of 32 feet per second per second.
From this hypothesis follows:
  (II) Every body starting from rest and freely falling towards, the Earth falls 16 t^2 feet in t seconds, whatever number t may be.
From II there follows in accordance with the logical principle permitting the application of a generalization to its instances, the infinite set of hypotheses:
  (IIIa) Every body starting from rest and freely falling for one second toward the Earth falls a distance of 16 feet.
  (IIIb) Every body starting from rest and freely falling for two seconds toward the Earth falls a distance of 64 feet. And so on.

In this deductive system the hypotheses at the second and third levels (II, IIIa, IIIb) follow from the one highest-level hypothesis (I); those at the third level (IIIa, IIIb) also follow from the one at the second level (II) (logically articulated structure).

The hypotheses in this deductive system are empirical general propositions with diminishing generality. The empirical testing of the deductive system is effected by testing the lowest-level hypotheses in the system. The confirmation or refutation of these is the criterion by which the truth of all hypotheses in the system are tested. The establishment of a system as a set of true propositions depends upon the establishment of its lowest-level hypotheses. E.g., when the distance in hypothesis III is not 16 feet, the hypothesis – and, therefore, the whole system – must be rejected.

Examples of deductive reasoning in medicine are hard to find. Eventually we found one presented as a logical (deductive) system. It is borrowed from Scandellari and Federspil (1977). They describe the 'thyroid' system:

(1) which patient with an autonomous thyroidal adenome has tachycardia? (explicandum);

(2) the thyroid gland produces a hormone capable of augmenting the cardiac pulse rate, if not otherwise diseased. This patient presents a thyroidal adenoma. This adenoma produces a raised amount of hormones (explanans);

(3) this patient has tachycardia because of a raised serum hormone level (conclusion).

The form looks the same as we recognize three levels of specification. The explicandum typically constitutes the general proposition, however, not a universal one. Not every patient with a thyroidal adenoma has signs of a fast cardiac pulserate. But we can assume a specific diagnostic classification with thyroidal adenomae and tachycardia. The explanations within the following level follow unmistakingly from the former level, specifying the particular cause of the tachycardia: the production of a hormone. However, a supernumerary hypothesis (if the heart is not otherwise diseased) is introduced. But to do this would be to make the observed facts evidence for a set of hypotheses which includes one which played no part in their deduction from the set, and would then make them indirect evidence for the supernumerary hypothesis and for its consequences. Since the supernumerary hypothesis might be any generalization whatever, this would have the undesirable result that any observable fact would be indirect evidence for any generalization whatever.

From the establishment that thyroid glands produce hormones capable of quickening the heart rate, does not unequivocally follow that a throidal adenoma produce hormones, and specifically a raised amount. The third level follows from the suppositions made in the second level. The process can easily be traced from bottom to top, but it requires foreknowledge as a prerequisite for this type of syllogism. Therefore, it falls short for the deductive reasoning process.

The problem with deductive inference in medicine arises to a great extent from the special situation with which medicine has to deal. Where in the lowest level a general proposition is applied to a special case (the application principle), the deduction of level II from level I is made by using integral causal relationships as laid down in medical knowledge itself. In other words, the derivation from level I to II is implicit to the medical knowledge. Regrettably, only a few of these kinds of logical derivations are possible in medicine, e.g., the attempts of Betacque and Gorry (1971) and de Vries Robbe (1978) in the field of nephropathology.

The derivation from level II to level III comes from a different source of knowledge. At this level empirical evidence, preferably numerical data, is required in order to proceed within this logical structure. For instance, in the thyroidal adenoma case we shall have to decide whether a particular pulserate is within or outside a 'normal' range. The notion of 'normality' requires an empirical knowledge which is mainly derived from statistical data. It is the conjunction of the two sources of knowledge which complicates medical problem-solving and might form an obstacle to the application of medical decision-making. It is our supposition that the differences between the two knowledge bases are not generally recognized, and in most conversation and discussion totally confused.

With a slight modification to Braithwaite (1968) we shall present a form of deductive reasoning with medical examples.

One of the main purposes in organizing scientific hypotheses into a deductive system is to make direct evidence for each lowest-level hypothesis indirect evidence for all other lowest-level hypotheses; although no amount of empirical evidence suffices to prove any of the hypotheses in the system, yet any piece of empirical evidence for any part of the system helps towards establishing the whole of the system. The ultimate testing of a hypothesis is against a particular case.

(I)   According to the evidence the underlying disease is of origin A (the pathophysiology of an organ or organ system). There is, e.g., a lung disease, or there is a hyperfunction of the thyroid gland). From this hypothesis follows.

(II)   The observed evidence (symptoms and signs) can only be explained by the B explanation of the A origin. The former disease can, e.g., only be explained by an inflammation of the lungs, the second by nervousness, weakness, sensitivity to heat, sweating, restless overcapacity, weight loss, tremor, palpitation, stare lid lag, and exophthalmus.

(IIIa) In case of B explanation there must be a C test of D level confirmative of the B (e.g., the demonstration of pneumococci in the sputum of the patient, or a raised blood level of thyroid hormone corresponding with a certain weight loss).

(IIIb) In case of B explanation there must be a C test of E level (E $\ddagger$ D) refutative of B (e.g., when micro-organisms of the origin Bact. pneumococci are demonstrated there cannot be an increasing antibody titre for a different micro-organism, or, a raised blood level of thyroid hormone is not a consequence of glycosuria in case of weight loss).

Tested against this particular case:

f_1:   In all cases of A disease the level D of test C is within the range R (e.g., above a certain number of micro-organisms, or, more than x pounds of weight loss).

g_1:   In this case the level D of the test C is within the range R.

We can easily trace the general propositions of levels I and II, typically based on medical knowledge. Level III represents the particular case on which two tests have to be performed: one for the confirmation and another for the falsification. As in all biological situations the outcomes of the tests are submitted to natural variation. By designing a particular range R we are able to decide upon its validity to this case. Clearly the establishment of the range is a matter of statistics; it cannot be deduced from medical knowledge. Where these two elements, medical knowledge and (medical) statistics, coincide decision-making can take place. That is, when, deductively, f_1 and g_1 coincide, we define a logical verification. However, this verification can still be false as a general proposition. However many conjunctions of f and g have been examined and found to confirm the hypothesis, there still will be unexamined cases in which the hypothesis might be false without contradicting any of the observed facts.

This situation is different if g_1 is observed to be false. The conjunction not-g_1 and f_1 is logically incompatible with the hypothesis being true; the hypothesis has to be refuted.

From the examples it may become clear that whereas in the pneumonia case there is some logical system, in the thyroid case this internal logic is absent. Not only there is no unambiguous explanation of the symptoms to the disease, there is also no obligatory weight loss in all cases of thyroidal hyperfunction. So it seems that a deductive system is not only case dependent but also subject to the state of medical knowledge. Where several underlying pathophysiological processes are unknown or partly known, it is hardly plausible that deductive systems will become the prevalent method of medical problem-solving in the near future.

Hypothetico-deductive reasoning

The hypothetico-deductive scheme of thought is meant to be an alternative to the inductive strategy. The term is misleading insofar as its purpose is to circumvent the imperfections of the inductive stratagem without drawing the full consequences of the deductive method. Hypothetico-deductive reasoning tries to combine the imaginative, creative act of hypothesis generation with the logically articulated structure of the deductive inference.

Medawar (1969) listed a number of positive features of this method. Whether these features were really observed in practice or form part of some wishful thinking was not communicated.

(1) A clear distinction is made between discovery (a creative thought) and justification or proof (in the sense of probation, the act or action of testing or trial), now resolved into two separate and dissociated episodes of thought.

(2) The initiative for the kind of action that is distinctively scientific is held to come, not from the apprehension of 'facts', but from an imaginative preconception of what might be true.

(3) The hypothetico-deductive scheme provides a theory of special in-

centive. Our observations no longer range over the universe of observables: they are confined to those that have a bearing on the hypothesis under investigation.

(4) It allows also for the continual rectification or running adjustment of hypotheses by the process of negative feedback.

(5) Error is simply explained – the fact that scientific research so very often goes wrong. Scientific error is now an ordinary part of human fallibility: we simply guess wrong, take a wrong view, form a mistaken opinion.

(6) Luck, unintelligible in inductive reasoning, now makes sense. The lucky accident fulfils a prior expectation, however vaguely formulated it may have been.

(7) The hypothetico-deductive scheme gives due weight to the critical purposes of experimentation: we carry out experiments more often to discriminate between possibilities than to enlarge the stockpile of factual information.

A strong argument for the hypothetico-deductive scheme is the separation of the creative act from its justification. In the inductive stratagem creation and justification are framed within one line of thought. When the creation (of hypotheses) is left aside, the act of justification is open to severe criticism. However, as justification no longer controls creation, imagination can generate an unlimited number of 'creative thoughts'. It opens the door to the fool who can ask more than ten wise men can answer. But, as Medawar argues, 'the hypotheses that enter our minds will as a rule be plausible and not, as in theory they could be, idiotic'. 'But this implies the existence of some internal censorship which restricts hypotheses to those that are not absurd, and the internal circuitry of this process is quite unknown'.

It is our supposition that this censorship must be appreciated as a mental state descending from the Baconian statement on 'unfamiliar thoughts' which can lead to a state of uncertainty (see section Methods in science). This impression would imply a severe limitation of the creative thought. It would limit the search for hypotheses to the pre-known, to our experience which determines the relevance we shall ascribe to the case at hand.

We are not so sure that a restricted hypothesis generation, restricted with regard to experiential knowledge, does not influence the act of proof. When this act is assumed to follow the ritual of deductive inference, the falsification of the generated idea is the logical implication. However, this presumes that our observations (eventually) will tend to falsify the hypothesis: or we may come to think that our observations may themselves have been faulty, or may have been made against a background of misconceptions: or our experiment(s) may have been badly designed.

It is very unlikely that individuals would reason in this way. It asks for a denial of their own observations, a reasoning process directed towards the falsification of their thoughts, as well as a reappraisal of their original standpoint; a standpoint which arises from their body of personal knowledge. In our opinion the schism between the creative and the justificatory act is an artificial one. Both the creative act and the procedure of proof control each other mutually, as is the case in inductive reasoning.

If a hypothesis is found to be false correction is obligatory. When do we know a hypothesis to be false? When a prediction arising from the conclusion of the inferential process, its logical output, cannot be verified by our experiment(s). This would lead to regulation by means of feedback, the control of performance by the consequences of the act performed. Reconsideration of the inference process must lead to the reconsideration of the original creative thought and even to refutation. But we are never sure that the experiment was correct or correctly performed. Feedback mechanisms are essential in scientific reasoning, but they ought to be part of a logical structure so that we can retrace our steps. The hypothetico-deductive method demands such a structure but man's commitment to standpoints as coming from personal knowledge and opinion makes refutation and corrective measures very unlikely to happen.

The hypothetico-deductive method tries to combine inductive and deductive reasoning into one scheme, but does not explain why this method should be preferred to the deductive inference process. It claims more freedom of the generative element, freedom for intuition to enter into the scientific process. But the meaning of intuition can vary relatively to the context in which it is placed. Deductive intuition is the instantly perceiving of logical implication from certain views. By force of logical reasoning it can bring us understanding and insight in phenomena in nature. Inductive intuition is like hitting on a sudden hypothesis, frequently a presumed relation between two or more events. The inference process is now directed at the demonstration of this co-existence. Even if this co-existence can be demonstrated, it does not explain, nor can it, the causes and backgrounds of the phenomena.

We follow Harre (1972) in his statement that in essence the hypothetico-deductive method is an inductive method. We shall continue by describing this latter method.

Inductive reasoning

We often say: 'Well, it is just plain logic!' in explaining some problem to another person, without realizing that our explanation is only our 'logical' interpretation of the problem. Obviously this type of 'logic' is different from the 'logic' in the deductive system. The common, daily 'logic' is a 'logic' stripped of nearly all the conditions, consequences and precautions that are attached to the deductive form. It expresses an insight, a firm belief in one's own statement, as being not only casual but of general importance also.

Inductive inferences are supposed to be based on observations, and the conclusions are more general than the observations on which they are based. E.g., 'red sky in the morning, shepherd's warning'. From having frequently observed the conjunction of two events (colour and weather) we feel compelled to assert a connection between them. As Hume pointed out, there is nothing other than 'habit' or 'custom' to justify induction. It has no logical warrant. In the 17th and 18th centuries, especially in the Anglo-Saxon sphere, inductive inference was supposed to provide *the* method of the empirical sciences. Philosophers such as Francis Bacon (1561–1626), and John Stuart Mill (1806–1873) formulated a variety of methods to secure its validity. Bacon visualized teams of people carrying out a multitude of experiments planned to embrace all possible enquiries which are relevant to the welfare of society. The experiments would yield a great mass of facts from which new, more general, laws of nature would be extracted by a process which is called 'induction'. In retrospect we can see that Bacon's 'new method' was not really a practical way of doing science; rather unkindly it has been called 'research by adminis-tration' (Brown, 1986).

However, both philosophers, Bacon and Mill, and their successors have strongly advocated this type of scientific reasoning. Although the principles of induction have been repudiated or allowed to fade away, we retain the impression that most of what is presented as 'scientific research' still bears the mark of induction.

What is induction? In its simplest form induction assures us that what is true of each must be true of all. It is arguing from the particular to the general. It always has to add something to reach a universal statement. Induction is, therefore, always ampliative in nature. 'Inductivism is a complex of beliefs of which the salient points are: Truth lies all around us in Nature, so that the scientist's main task is to discern and record matters of fact and then to classify and appraise them according to certain more or less well-defined rules – whereupon the Truth will certainly reveal itself.' (Medawar, 1975).

And, indeed, what is more appealing than looking about one and observe, and while observing the hypotheses as universal laws of nature come to you all by themselves. But the 'habit of mind' also makes us believe that we can predict things on the mere ground of assumed foreknowledge and similarity. It is far from obvious, from a logical point of view, that we are justified in inferring universal statements from singular ones, no matter how numerous; for any conclusion drawn in this way may always turn out to be false; no matter how many white swans we may have observed, this does not justify the conclusion that all swans are white (Popper, 1959).

Nevertheless, the prediction that the next swan we will see will be a white one, can momentarily fulfil the demands of plausibility, our reasonable belief. It is in this direction that philosophers have created conditions to strengthen the method and conclusions of induction. An important exponent of the inductive method is John Stuart Mill. He created 'Mill's canons' (as described by Harre (1972), of which the most important are:

(I) the canon of agreement: if two or more instances of the phenomenon under investigation have only one circumstance in common, the cir-cumstance in which alone all the instances agree is the cause (or effect) of the given phenomenon. For example, if patients suffering from an infectious disease have the same bacteria in common, the particular bacteria is assumed to be the cause of this specific infectious disease.

(II) the canon of difference: if an instance in which the phenomenon under investigation occurs, and an instance in which it does not occur has every circumstance in common save one, the one occurring only in the former, i.e., the circumstance in which alone the two instances differ, is the effect, or the cause, or an indispensable part of the cause of the phenomenon. E.g., if two depressive patients, both from the same types of family and social background, differ in their marriage relation, this relation is assumed to be the cause or the effect of the depression.

The method of agreement stands on the ground that whatever can be eliminated is not connected with the phenomenon by any law. The method of difference has for its foundation that whatever cannot be eliminated is connected with the phenomenon by a law: these two main canons Mill offers us as the principles or among.the principles of inductive reasoning, for, having found the cause we have found the law, or so he thinks. Here are principles by which we can pass from facts to general laws.

These canons illustrate the typical character of inductive reasoning: the first canon stands for a heuristic search programme eliminating those symptoms and signs which are not consistent with an *a priori* statement. The second canon tests this statement for internal consistency in order to confirm it. When there is more than one causal factor, one has to do another experiment, with the exclusion of one (or more) of the factors involved.

In a way it also illustrates the circular reasoning in inductive inference, especially when there are more than two factors involved, which is often the case in medicine. Recapitulating the process:

(1) there is a early hypothesis generation predominantly based on (assumed) analogies, as derived from the personal knowledge (mainly based on experience) of the actor;

(2) a heuristic search programme is performed looking for observational data consistent with the early hypothesis;

(3) as mixing of testing data and acquisition of new data takes place, both types of data can judge a hypothesis as well as generate a new one;

(4) because hypotheses arise from personal knowledge and belief, commitment to the hypotheses makes rejection improbable;

(5) the final choice is predominantly based on satisfying minimum-adjusted personal standards and the actor's feelings of certainty.

Furthermore, the Baconian statement about unfamiliar thoughts implies the existence of some internal censorship which restricts hypotheses to those that are not absurd.

Harre listed the arguments of inductivism into three principles.

(1) The principle of accumulation: augmenting knowledge to an existing knowledge base does not alter the latter. This principle is crucial for the plausibility of inductivism, although, generally speaking, it is hard to find arguments to maintain the principle. As we shall discuss in the next paragraph, this principle is equally important in the inductive probability theory.

(2) The principle of induction: inference of laws from accumulated singular facts can lead to the inference of true laws. The laws of nature are the codified and generalized facts. In modern science the operation of this principle is often seen in the effort to obtain numerical data and then

find (mathematical, statistical, etc.) functions to express them.

(3) The principle of instance confirmation: our belief in the degree of plausibility of (or our degree of belief in) a law is proportional to the number of instances that have been observed of the phenomenon described in the law. Everybody knows that in some experiments, e.g., tossing coins, the probability of casting heads or tails is 50%. However, when heads come up over and over again, many people are certaintly inclined to reconsider that estimation.

The concepts of inductive reasoning are so familiar to us that we hardly recognize them as factors or rules that we implicitly apply. Inductive reasoning is our daily, routine way of thinking; it is the 'habit' or 'custom' of mind.

Sage (1981) listed some of the concepts inductive people employ. The concepts:

(a) are drawn from personal experiences;
(b) involve elementary classification and generalization concerning tangible and familiar thoughts;
(c) involve direct cause and effect relationships, typically in simple two-variable situations;
(d) can be taught or understood by analogy, algorithms, effects, standard operating policy, or recipe;
(e) are 'closed' in the sense of not demanding exploration of possibilities outside the known environment of the perceived or stated data.

If we want to recapitulate the method of inductivism in one word we come up with: conservatism.

In all concepts and phrases in inductive reasoning there is not one real incentive for change, for disprove or discrediting, for reconsideration of steps already taken, for admitting a theory, a concept, a policy, etc., to be false, or at least to allow it to be submitted to serious tests. Because, can we not say with Nietzsche: 'Everything that reaches consciousness is utterly and completely adjusted, simplified, schematized, and interpreted'. In inductivism everything that comes to our mind is only submitted to verification, the verification of what we already think. When the verification process comes to an end we are quite relieved to find our statement justified, maybe on minimal grounds. It gives us the feeling, yes, the certainty, of being right. It provides us with the smell of truth. It strengthens our beliefs, it gives us that particular kind of security that must guide our steps in real life. It leaves no place for reconsideration, for contemplation of alternatives, because we know for sure that we are right. Rejection of hypotheses is not an innate characteristic feature of inductivism.

It does not mean that inductive judgements may not be true, for they may very well be true, and can serve as a guide in action, but they cannot be shown to be true. The fact that it works tells us little about its truth, it just tells us that it works, and the explanation why it works may be very different from what we think it is (Brehmer, 1980). The knowledge which can be learned from that particular experiment, therefore, adds nothing to the existing knowledge. It allows people to make mistakes and errors even after having provided them with substantial contra-evidence. Erasmus (1469–1536) provides us in his most famous book, 'The Pride of Folly', with a considerable number of examples of straight reasoning notwithstanding available (contra-)evidence. In our time, Tuchman (1984) gives in her entertaining book, 'The March of Folly', an historical survey of a number of the world's greatest follies in political decision-making.

Mankind has inhabited the Earth for many thousands of years, but for the most basic functions, humanity and understanding, hardly anything is changed. Obviously we prefer our certainty of living in a maladjusted world to anything that can bring human co-omunity to a profound re-orientation.

Scientists hope to contribute to knowledge and understanding. It is our purpose to elucidate a number of features that can be met in clinical practice. Inductive reasoning might be one of those features.

Probabilistic reasoning

The number of techniques for analysing data has increased enormously over the past decades. These techniques are almost all based on probability theory, and they have been developed so as to end up with some kind of inference, some statement about the real world. The concept of probability, however, is rather abstract and hence the question arises: what is the interpretation of the notion of probability in real world situations? In answering this question we reach the foundations of probability theory and, as is the case in many sciences, it is precisely here that differences in opinion appear. The foundations of this concept have been the object of much discussion. Different interpretations have resulted in different axiomatic systems.

It is a mistake to believe that the word 'probability' has only one important meaning: actually it has various meanings. We shall in this paragraph follow the usual distinction:

(I)   objective probability; and

(II) subjective probability (also named: inductive probability)

The former meaning refers to the mathematical type of probability, or the statistical probability. In its simplest form it can be defined as 'the relative frequency of an event 'a' occurring within a reference class (also called 'population') 'b'. Put into a formula it runs as

$$p\,(a,\,b) = r$$

where 'a' given 'b' is also called the "conditional probability of a under 'b'; and 'r' is some fraction between 0 and 1 (these limits included). Sometimes another formula is denoted, running as

$$p\,(a) = r$$

or, the (absolute) probability of 'a' being 'r'. This 'absolute' probability of 'a' has sometimes been called the 'prior' or 'a $priori$' probability. As these latter terms are frequently encountered in the literature on decision analysis, they are mentioned here.

The 'absolute' probability, however, is scarcely to be understood, except in a trivial way when a specific reference class is taken as 'understood'. For there is no point in saying 'malaria is a common disease' unless you specify 'in tropical areas'. In the same way, the expression $p(D)$, the 'absolute' probability of having a disease D, cannot have any relevance within the framework of objective (statistical) probability, unless a conditional reference class is taken as understood or will subsequently be added.

This reference class 'b' has to be defined in finite terms, as can be shown in the next example. The statement $p(a) = r$ asserts that among the 'n' elements of the sample 'nr' elements have the property 'a' (when 'p' is defined by the frequency with which a certain element occurs within a total population of elements: $p = n_1/n$). Suppose that 'n' belongs to an infinite universe of elements, than the meaning of $p(a) = r$ becomes highly obscure, it will be indeterminate, for $n = \infty$

Suppose we have some, more or less definite, idea about the possibility that the patient has disease D. The conditional reference class in that case is: 'my medical knowledge', 'my experience'. In those cases we can take for granted only that the condition is subjectively determined.

When I ask students to estimate the chance of getting a six when in casting a dice, the answer (almost) invariably is: 1/6. The second question is: 'What are your estimates upon getting a six in the next cast?' The answer (almost) invariably is: 1/6. However, this is an erroneous answer. Because, in the case of the next cast I was only interested in getting a six. So my reference class consists of a six or a non-six; the chance, therefore, is 1/2. The students implicitly incorporate the condition: 'for an infinite number of casts'.

Two other assumptions have been made. First, the scattering of events is random; this is an essential prerequisite for experiments with limited numbers. This can easily be shown when we denote for a six a 1 and for non-six 0. When the following sequence of six's and non-six's comes up

00000000000000000010000000000000000000000000110000000000001000

evidently the six's and the non-six's are not randomly scattered in the series of casts. The chance of touching upon a sample of non-six's is, in this limited case, much greater than in a more equal distribution.

Secondly, it is assumed that the circumstances do not change, e.g., by changing the dice for a loaded one. That does not necessarily exclude probability theory, but it leads to a totally different experiment.

Apparently, a number of conditions has to be fulfilled for rational application of objective probability theory.

The case of the next cast is an example of subjective (or inductive) probability. In that case one has to define a virtual or conceivable sequence of events. In asking for the chance on the next toss a probability value of the form '$p' (a,b)$' is assigned to a single event as a representative of the virtual sequence of events. It demands for the definition of the condition(s) which would determine this virtual sequence; the conditions that produce the, as called after Popper, hidden propensity; the hidden propensity that would give the single case a numerical probability. This matter is especially valid in subjective expected utility theory, as we shall meet in the chapter on clinical decision-making.

In medicine we are specifically interested in subjective probability for we wish to know if a particular patient is suffering from that particular disease given those symptoms. If we were able to assign a numerical value to this pi ibability it would be helpful to the doctor in establishing a diagnosis and a the rapeutic policy.

The formulae look the same but they represent, nevertheless, different meanings: a meaning in objective probability theory and another in subjective probability theory.

Conditions for the valid application of the probability theory

Von Mises made a substantial contribution by defining the conditions relevant to the frequency approach in probability theory. These conditions are known as Von Mises' axioms which run as follow.
 (1) 'Random' experiment in finite sequences. Definition: a random (or chance) phenomenon is an empirical phenomenon characterized by the property that its observation under a given set of circumstances does not always lead to the same observed outcome (so that there is no deterministic regularity) but rather to different outcomes in such a way that there is statistical regularity. By this is meant that numbers exist between 0 and 1 that represent the relative frequency with which the different possible outcomes may be observed in a series of observations of independent occurrences of the phenomenon.
 (2) A 'random' experiment implies 'stable' relative frequencies (a more or less regular, equable scattering of properties). But these frequencies depend on 'n' (the number of events). The empirically established fact that relative frequencies stabilize in long sequences of trials is of utmost importance because it has become the basis of a frequency definition of probability.
 (3) The impossibility of a winning gambling system. To put it differently, we study sequences which are 'unpredictable' or 'random'.
 People often deny this requirement. People are very much inclined to assume orderly patterns where, actually, randomness is the case. Most gamblers assume some kind of order in roulette, many people predict that an observed trend will continue in the future. All this implies a reference to a type of orderly patterns which such events can simulate only by coincidence. This raises the question whether orderliness is merely a coincidence or a man-made assumption. If our appraisal of order is an act of personal knowledge, so is the assessment of probability to which it is allied. This is, of course, quite evident when the ordered pattern is contrived by ourselves (Polanyi, 1958).
 Probability, according to Von Mises, can, therefore, be defined as the limit of relative frequency in a collective (this term will be defined in the

next condition). Polanyi's statement about orderliness refers to this axiom, but differs in the sense of personal imposed orderliness versus the coincidental randomness to be overcome by assuming unlimited boundaries.

These conditions lead to the following definition of a collective.

(4) A collective is a long sequence of identical observations, each observation leading to a definite numerical result, provided that the sequence fulfils the two conditions: existence of 'stable' frequencies and 'randomness'.

As can be inferred from this definition, Von Mises replaces the infinite sequences condition by a finite one. Within the finite sequence of reasonably long extension it also defines the limiting frequencies and the randomness. It sets the conditions for samples as they are drawn from their parent populations. Probability calculus teaches us to compute the probability distributions in derived collectives from given distributions in the collectives from which they have been derived. By means of four operations (place selection, mixing, partition, and combining) the new collective can be derived from a given one (de Leene and Koerts).

However, is there any possibility of drawing logical conclusions about the relative frequencies when the distributions in the collective(s) are largely unknown, as is often the case? To this end, in our opinion, two rules have been implicitly introduced.

(a) An event with a very low probability of occurrence will not occur at an individual trial; and

(b) All probability properties (e.g., distribution functions) are introduced *a priori*.

In a frequentistic, or statistical, sense the first rule is often, implicitly, applied. This situation can be compared with a lottery: if the number of winning tickets is small in comparison with the total number of tickets (low relative frequency), it is thought to be impossible for any ticket to be a winning one. Nevertheless, there must be some winning ticket. Von Mises' axioms restrict the domain to the application of mass phenomena (law of large numbers). However, surveying medical research has taught that rapid convergence commonly exists, i.e., sample sizes seem to approach very rapidly the possible sizes.

Bayes' theorem, as a law of large numbers, seems to solve the problem because roughly speaking it says: 'If, in one set of observations, 'n' being a large number, the relative frequency of success (positive outcomes) is equal to 'q', then we expect *with great certainty* that 'p' is equal to 'q.' This means that in the derived collective (say our sample size) the majority of elements possess an inferred probability value close to the relative frequency value (n_1/n).

But logically nothing can be concluded about a specific element 'a' out of the collective, for the theory admits the possibility that 'a' with the probability value 'p' deviates substantially from the relative frequency value. This can partially be overcome by creating a large 'n', especially when the prior distribution (e.g., the number of black or white marbles in the bag, the number of patients with disease X in a population) is unknown.

Suppose that we have taken all the precautions to define a correct collective, we still can run into problems like:

(1) all probability properties (e.g., distribution functions) must be introduced *a priori*. In medicine they are usually unknown;

(2) the number of observations must be (very) large (which is usually impossible to achieve in medicine);

(3) increase of numbers is usually impossible because of changing situations, time limits, or because of ethical obstacles;

(4) following these instructions we have constructed procedures which normally lead to solutions which are consistent with the *a priori* assumptions. We are also creating the circular reasoning of self-fulfilment, the inductive inference process. And there is no way of knowing whether or not we are far from reality.

One other condition as defined in Von Mises' axioms has to be discussed: independence. This most important element, also mentioned in Bayes' doctrine of chances, is often overlooked or brushed aside by ambitious decision analysts. As we have argued, the testing of a hypothesis is an integral part of a reasoning process whether that process is deductive or inductive. The probabilistic hypothesis predicts that a singular event has a certain tendency to be realized. This prediction can be tested by repeating the experiment under the conditions prescribed. It is obvious that the relative frequencies of the results within the sequence of repeated tests are equal to unity (or nearly so). In other words, when the frequency distributions differ largely from one experiment to its subsequent one, test results will say next to nothing about the plausibility of the hypothesis. It is, therefore, absolutely essential for a repetition of an experiment that each repetition occurs under the same standard conditions. But this means that in an experimental set-up, the earlier experiments must *not* affect the later ones. For otherwise the later ones operate under new conditions. The experiments must be *independent* (see Popper, 1983).

One can easily guess that these situations, i.e., independence of tests, are created only (very) rarely. As (patho)biological processes affect human beings as well as (courses of) diseases, we can hardly imagine how to fulfil this independency condition. Nevertheless, it is a major condition in order to come to valid and reliable probabilistic statements.

As mentioned in Chapter I, in subjective probability the two main sources of knowledge, the pathological/pathophysiological and the (medical) statistical one, come together. Within subjective probability theory the formula '$p(a, b) = r$' means that we assert a certain probability about a particular element 'a' under the condition 'b' = 'all our relevant knowledge'. As we discussed in the former paragraph, the inference from level I (general statement) to level II (intermediate) is based on our knowledge of patho-(physio)logical processes. It enables us to create or to perform experiments which can decide upon the specific hypothesis. It may be clear that when the condition of 'b' is next to zero the total result will be undetermined.

But here we meet one of the weaknesses of subjective probability calculus: it depends on personal knowledge. The outcome can only express the degree of belief a certain person assigns to a certain proposition; it cannot be generalized across situations and persons. This problem brings us to the implications of probability theory.

Logical implications of probability theory

Subjective (or inductive) probability measures the strength of support given to a hypothesis (h) by the evidence (e). In the notation of Carnap (1960) it takes the form

$$C\,(h,\ e) = r$$

which is the degree of confirmation (C) of 'h' on the basis of 'e'; or, the quantified subjective probability is the degree of credence an individual X accords to a hypothesis 'h' being given the evidence 'e'.

The hypothesis may be any statement of a future event. Any set of known or assumed facts may serve as evidence; it consists usually of the results of observations which have been made. In this sense, inductive probability theory, as it is developed by Carnap, is a principle of learning from experience which guides, or rather ought to guide, all inductive thinking in everyday affairs and in science. It expresses in quantitative terms our confidence in the outcome of a particular process (Carnap, 1960).

The degree of confirmation (C) is sometimes reflected in a fair betting quotient, and studied as such. To say, e.g., that the hypothesis 'h' has the probability 'p' (say 3/5) with respect to the evidence ('e'), means that to anyone to whom only this evidence but no other relevant knowledge is available (the principle of 'fair bet'), it would be reasonable to believe in 'h' to the degree 'p' or, more exactly, it would be unreasonable for him to bet on 'h' at odds higher than '$p/(1-p)$' (in the example 3:2). A probabilistic diagnosis is such a 'fair bet system'.

As stated before, this kind of probability must be understood in the context of a virtually defined sequence of events. If we want to know the outcome of a proposed action, or the plausibility that a next toss will be heads we have to assume an orderly trend. However, an orderly trend is contradicted by the objective probability theory, as we learned from Von Mises' axioms.

Inductive probability can be defined as a way of judging hypotheses concerning unknown events. In order to be reasonable this judging must be guided by our knowledge of observed events. More specifically, other things being equal, a future event is to be regarded as the more probable, the greater the relative frequency of similar events observed so far under similar circumstances.

It seems plausible in daily practice, that from the observation of what has in former instances been the consequence of a certain cause of action, one may make a judgement as to what is likely to be the consequence of that cause of action another time; and that the larger the number of experiments we have to support a conclusion, the more reason we have to take it for granted. Our confidence that a certain therapy will work in a present case of a certain disease is the higher the more frequently it has worked in past cases.

Objective interpretations assume that the probability depends solely upon similar conditions (repetitive experiments), whereas subjective interpretations depend upon the state of our knowledge, or of our beliefs. In the words of the formula '$p\ (a,\ b) = r$' the 'subjectivist' takes 'a' as the basis for testing, while the 'objectivist' refers to 'r' as the basis for testing. If we replace the Carnapian formula '$C\ (h,\ e) = r$' for the more general '$p\ (a,\ b) = r$', we have to realize that the main difference between the objective probability and the subjective probability is in the 'b'. In objective probability it defines the conditions with which repetitive experiments have to take place; in the subjective probability it is a measure of our own imperfect knowledge (were we to have perfect knowledge, the outcome should always be certain!). In objective probability it is essential to keep the 'b' constant; in subjective probability the 'b' changes all the time as the result of our changing knowledge (under the condition that we shall learn something, positive or negative, from any experiment, say a patient case).

The claim has been made that the outcomes of the various types of probability are interchangeable. This notion comes from the theory that value assignment in subjective probability comes from 'fair betting'. A model of 'fair betting' is given in Carnap's example. The question, however, is whether this mode is always applied. Fair betting is assumed to be repetitive. It is mainly based upon a rough questionnaire method which aims at subsuming every case under a very large class. It takes only a minimal amount of property characteristics into account as a huge class of repetitions have to be built. It consciously neglects available relevant information to avoid the construction of more specified classes with smaller numbers. This is due to the fact that 'b' is considered as defining repetitive experimental conditions. The more specific, the more individual characteristics which are involved, the smaller the classes which, therefore, approach numbers that cannot fulfil the Von Mises' axioms. They fall within the category of gambling.

The results of gambling calculations as disregarding objective probability conditions have been shown by Feller (quoted in Popper, 1983) for a red – blue game with an objective chance distribution of 50%. Disregarding the independence condition produced observed frequencies that were 1/6 and 5/6 instead of the actual 1/2!

It means that replacing probability estimates from research in (diseased) populations into formula valid for subjective (inductive) probability is very hazardous. It creates one of the more difficult problems to be solved in medical decision-making. If one is not aware of differences between the two types of probability, decision-making can produce outcomes far-removed from reality, apart from the variations due to the personal knowledge and backgrounds of the physicians.

In (medical) decision-making, nevertheless, the calculation of the probability estimates may direct the choice between alternative hypotheses and choosing among a number of possible actions. The choice is to be determined by a comparison of the desirable effects of believing one hypothesis if it is true and the undesirable effects of believing it if it is false with the desirable and undesirable effects of believing the other hypothesis if it is true or false; commonly described as true and false positives and negatives. The criteria for this choice will be in terms of the arithmetical relationships of four values – the gain or loss obtained by choosing one hypothesis if it is true or false respectively, the gain or loss by choosing the other hypothesis if it is true or false respectively. The different assignments of these four values will give different choices (Braithwaite, 1968).

The numerical values come from extrapolation: the calculation of probabilities which are not given from probabilities which are given. However, this type of calculation only gives rise to subjective interpretations. It treats the degree of probability as a measure of the feelings of certainty or uncertainty, or belief or doubt, which may be aroused in us by certain assertions or conjectures.

The degree of confirmation only expresses the degree of belief, the degree of certainty a physician has in his own inference and conclusions. This belief is, by virtue of the lack of an objective reference, mainly based upon his personal experience and his personal conceptions about health and disease. His conclusions only resemble the proximity of the singular statement to his personal knowledge and conceptions but tells us nothing about the real situation. There cannot be a plausible reason to treat inductive conclusions (e.g., medical diagnoses) otherwise than as preliminary hypotheses which can only be accepted as objective knowledge (and, therefore calculable and teachable) when they are submitted to severe tests.

This raises two questions: 'does the medical process permit such testing?' and 'will the conclusion of a medical process always be a provisional expression of the doctor's belief about a patient?'.

It leaves us with the inductivist's claim that inductive probability can guide us in our learning from experience. Although the stabilization of 'r' by accumulating knowledge from experienced cases cannot be doubted, still a number of objections can be raised. When 'r' approximates or equals 'n_1/n', 'n' being the total number of observations and 'n_1' those that favourably contribute to our knowledge, the formula becomes:

$$p\,(a,\ b) = r \approx n_1/n.$$

If 'n' grows (very) large, then any new observation will have very little influence upon 'r', because the quotient $(n_1 + 1)/(n + 1)$ will be almost the same as 'n_1/n'. It is, in a statement of Popper (1983), 'a thinking of diminishing returns'. Besides, it also poses an unfavourable result. It shows, as is the claim of inductive probability theory, that this theory of learning attributes an immense authority to our past. After a lifetime of learning (and perhaps much less than that) there can be no hope for learning more: the authority of our past experience makes a revision practically impossible. In other words, the older we get, the more rusty, the more sluggish we get, being tied down by the past; and the same must hold for science' (Popper, 1983).

It also leaves aside the possibility of the processing of incorrect data. As subjective probability theory must rely on personal knowledge, it is very hard to establish whether anything can logically be deduced from the applications of this theory. As it is the method of choice in medical decision-making, we assume that there are several problems still waiting for a solution.

(For a more profound discussion on this matter we recommend the writings of, *interalia*, Braithwaite, Carnap, Harre, Keynes, Lakatos, and Popper.)

Summary

'Science' is not that universal discipline that I used to know. Controversies are marring the scene. It was my idea to compare the characteristics of the method of science with those of the problem-solving methods of practising physicians. It turned out to be a difficult idea. Three methods of scientific reasoning can be distinguished, all three claiming to be the most creative, elegant, efficient, proficient and reliable strategy guiding to the universal truth; the truth being that particular law in nature which reveals and explains whatever can be observed in nature. However, it seemed that the line between a general law and a personal belief in a statement is very small, and often confused.

The supporters of the two rival schools of scientific reasoning made themselves very clear in their discussions. The strict and rigid scheme of the deductive reasoning is the most rational but also the most laborious method. By its strict conditions and rules this strategy is the most consistent and explanatory method; especially when the falsification condition is incorporated. However, as a practical and handy way to solve problems it lacks flexibility and speed. For minor problems like those physicians encounter in their daily work, the deductive method seems hardly suitable. For this purpose the inductive strategy seems to be more appropriate. Though it misses the rigid rules and conditions, it leads certainly to quick conclusions and outcomes. Regrettably, these outcomes have not always the quality that should be required in science. Although the supporters of inductive logic (e.g., Carnap[3]) assert differently, we follow Popper (1959, 1983) in stating that induction can never lead to a true explanation of what is in need of explanation. By mixing the act of hypothesis generation with the act of its justification the reasoning tends to be circular and conducive to the confirmation of the pre-established standpoint, that which was pre-known.

The hypothetico-deductive strategy suggests a distinction between the hypothesis generation episode and that of its proof. In our opinion these two episodes are so greatly interconnected that separation seems implausible. In theory it could be possible, but in practice it must fail as a result of human behaviour. In trying to circumvent the disadvantages of the inductive method and avoid the laborious and difficult deductive strategy, its originators forgot to demarcate this method from the others.

To evaluate the inductive inference process probability theory was in-

---

[3] See, e.g., Carnap, R. in: Lakatos: *Inductive Logic*, 1968.

troduced. The strict rules of mathematical statistics certainly marshalled the process and enhanced the validity of its conclusions. However, the limitations of the probability theory made clear that the territory of its application is restricted. Especially in the clinical sphere with its limited numbers of observable elements (patients) the contribution of probability theory to medical research is rather small.

Even if 'science' is not a uniform, unambiguous and universal discipline its study was worthwhile and allowed for the creation of models which could serve the purpose of this study.

Chapter III

Human thinking and problem-solving and their relationship to medicine

> Another error is an impatience of doubts and haste to assertion without due and mature suspension of judgments. If a man will begin with certainty, he shall end in doubts, but if he will begin in doubts he shall end in certainties.
>
> F. Bacon

Introduction

Human thinking processes have been the subject of many theories and philosophies, from the earliest days of mankind to the present day, from Socrates to Artificial Intelligence. Yet, we have only a diffuse picture of their true nature. First, the ancient Greek philosophers (Plato, Aristotle) gave shape to theories about human thinking and reasoning, followed by philosophers like Locke, Bacon, Kant, Descartes and Mill in later days. New incentives came from a different discipline, experimental psychology, which was founded by Wilhelm Wundt (1832–1890) at the University of Leipzig and followed by psychologists from the University of Wuerzburg. They applied 'introspective methods' to higher mental processes. After the demise of the Wuerzburg school, most thinking processes were studied under the guise of 'problem-solving'. Under the influence of economic principles (utilitarian theory, J. S. Mill, 1806–1873) and game theory (Von Neumann, 1928) a new branch on this tree appeared: decision theory, which is mainly preoccupied with the outcomes of the thinking processes.

With all these developments one is now confronted with the problem of information inundation rather than information scarcity. There being nothing definite, it is especially difficult to choose from among the plethora of publications in order to present the reader with a relevant and concise survey about the theories of reasoning, problem-solving and decision-making. Therefore, controversies and personal interpretations cannot be avoided, especially when particular applications to medical processes are made.

Although human thinking processes, problem-solving and decision-making are branches of the same tree, they differ in their background and scope so that there is good reason to discuss each of these items separately.

In contrast to animals human beings are capable of creative thinking. It enables them to solve problems beyond the basic needs of their own survival. Our thinking enables us to gain insight into the processes of nature, discover orderliness and natural laws, and to help our fellowmen. However, our physical thinking capabilities, (our mind), have placed barriers to the handling of information. Our minds can only process small amounts of information at a time. In other words, there is a limited entry to the immense storage capacity in which our memories reside.

The interesting question, in our opinion, is how humans can overcome these limitations, as we obviously digest large amounts of information at a time. There must be some tricks to overcome this limitation; there have to be openings to pass the barrier in order to have as free an entry as possible to our nearly unlimited memory. Cognitive studies have revealed interesting processes in human thinking. It is our strongly held opinion that these processes and methods influence the possibilities for creative thinking, information processing and problem-solving.

These general methods can certainly be attributed to the practising physician. However, studies in this field have been scarce. This can partly be ascribed to the task-environment (medical practice) as well as to the special nature of medical knowledge. The medical practice plays its particular role as it is placed between patients and their social and cultural environments, on one side, and the official medical knowledge on the other. Physicians have to balance between these two worlds. It affects their problem-solving and clinical judgements. It appeals to their abilities of creative thinking, their capabilities of processing information, and to the correct and adequate application of their knowledge whether it is acquired from 'official' textbooks or from experience. It is not surprising when these two worlds sometimes clash and lead to sub-optimal problem-solving.

Human cognition and the development of thought

The main preoccupation of epistemology or the theory of cognition, (which is the philosophical approach to human thinking), was and is the method of cognition: 'How do we know that we actually see what we see', and the truthfulness of the observation: 'How do we know that what we see is true, is certain'. The Platonian view is that what we see is in reality a foreshadow of our world of ideas and conception, while Aristotle considered our world of cognition as an impression and depiction of the world around us. In the former conception the truth must come forth by collecting personal opinions and attitudes, and by inducing a general statement from them, as truth can only be found in the human being itself. In the Aristotelian view truth can only be deduced by bringing conceptions into relation with observable facts. Only facts can verify or refute the man-made conceptions as truth can only be found in nature itself.

However, human beings seldom follow rules of sound reasoning in their search for the truth. Besides, as the truth sometimes can be frightening, they often comfort themselves with feelings of certainty instead of truthfulness. Doubts, lack of confidence, uncertainty about the truthfulness of observable facts, events, or objects, make people grasp at less optimal methods of decison-making. Besides, do we know where we can find the truth? Do we find it in ourselves as some kind of personal belief, or can we make truth objective by the force of logical deduction? It is especially these questions that have been stated in the philosophy of science and have given rise to heated debates between the adherents of both camps (see, e.g., Lakatos, 1968).

When a patient asks his doctor for the truth about his condition the doctor can try to find confirmation by testing the hypothesis against the evidence already acquired, or search his memory for an analogy of a similar case he has met before. However, what is the truth for the patient depends on the quality of the medical knowledge, its consistency and dependability; it depends on the medical knowledge of the physician; it also depends on what the physician views as the truth, and, last but not least, it depends on the method of inference the doctor employs.

As we have discussed above, the understanding of medical knowledge is crucial for the patient's question. In the Hippocratic view medical knowledge can only be explained within the context of the patient-physician contact. This type of knowledge relies heavily on the doctor's own experience. In the Galenic version medical knowledge is a scientific discipline, explaining the various patho(physio)logical relationships which can be observed among patients presenting equal or nearly equal symptom configurations.

The doctor's opinion about truth depends partly on his understanding of medical knowledge and partly on his inference strategy, the way he solves the problem. Problem-solving depends, among others, on the human capacity to process information and its adequate storage.

Problem-solving

Problem-solving enables mankind to react and respond to needs, to behave adequately and to survive in an environment that represents unpredictable threats and opportunities. Varying problems in changing environments require adequate processes to find adequate solutions. Are these qualities inherited or acquired?

The excellent studies by Piaget (1977) reveal much of the phases of thinking processes in children. The author distinguishes 4 stages of thought and reasoning:

(1)   the sensory-motor stage of early childhood; the child reacts directly to the stimuli of his sensory organs;

(2)   the preoperatory stage: the younger child tries to discover the world without being goal-directed;

(3)   the concrete operations stage: here we enter the stage of the school-child. The child is already capable of certain logical reasoning processes but only to the extent of applying particular operations to concrete objects or events in the immediate present;

(4)   the stage of formal operations: the principal novelty of this period is the capacity to reason in terms of verbally stated hypotheses and no longer merely in terms of concrete objects and their manipulations. This is a

decisive turning point, because to reason hypothetically and to deduce the consequences that the hypotheses necessarily imply (independent of the intrinsic truth or falseness of the premises) is a normal reasoning process. Hypothetical reasoning implies the subordination of the real to the realm of the possible, and consequently the linking of all possibilities to one another by necessary implications that encompass the real, but at the same time go beyond it. The individual who becomes capable of hypothetical reasoning, by reason of that very fact, will take an interest in problems that go beyond his immediate field of experience. Propositional logic appears to be one of the essential conquests of formal thought. This fourth period can no longer be characterized as a proper stage, but would already seem to be a structural advancement in the direction of specialization. This stage is reached in different areas at different ages according to aptitude and professional specialization. It can only develop after the scheme of causality has been firmly established, approximately around the ages of 12 to 15 years.

In the third stage the notion of order and causality is developed. Through this kind of reasoning the child is able to connect not only concrete objects but concrete events also. Moreover, through the observation of co-occurrence of two (or more) events he can learn some basic principles of causality. From a particular co-occurrence he can infer that the occurrence of event A is followed, or will be followed, by event B; and from this he can reason what the cause might be. This type of reasoning implies the notion of order. The notion of chance or probability is developed in the next stage. The notion of chance needs a higher level of reasoning because probabilism contrasts with the schema of order and causal thinking.

Piaget and Inhelder made their observations and studies in privileged schools in Geneva and Lausanne (Switzerland). It is assumed that the populations of these schools are not really representative of the general population. We suppose that not everyone enters the fourth stage of formal operations, the stage in which logic and probabilism is developed. Smedslund (1966) maintains that Piaget and Inhelder's stages of development represent different levels of cognitive functioning at which adults operate. Thus, although adults are capable of using disconfirming information for the inferring of relationships, they frequently fail to do so and operate at a lower, more frequently used level, for example, concrete reasoning. At the concrete-operatory level a structure cannot be generalized to different heterogenous contents but remains attached to a system of objects or the properties of these objects. A formal structure seems, in contrast, to be capable of generalization as it deals with hypotheses. It cannot be stressed enough that by disregarding the thought levels of operation experimental studies may lead to largely varying results and hence conclusions.

It is especially in medicine with its individual-oriented approach that there will always be the possibility of sticking to the concrete-operatory level, as Smedslund predicts. It incorporates the danger of asserting or predicting much more than the evidence conveys. It can be prevented by training and using the more imaginative formal-operational thought.

People who have been trained in the employment of formal operational thought, are able to use concepts which

(1) are hypothetical and based on alternative scenarios which may be contrary to the facts: the generated hypotheses or ideas may be contradicted by the facts;

(2) are 'open-ended' in the sense of requiring speculation about unstated possibilities;

(3) require deductive reasoning using unverified and perhaps flawed hypotheses;

(4) require a theory to be devised which is often not directly related to the original concept or discipline. This theory might be developed by other concepts or from other disciplines which may have only a remote connection to the original concept. For instance, studying physicians' problem-solving behaviour by means of theories from cognitive psychology, information theory, philosophy, etc.;

(5) require the definition of the theory as sketched in (4), and the identification and structuring of intermediate concepts not initially specified (Sage, 1981).

However, a big step is required to pass from concrete-operatory reasoning to formal operational thought.

Thought processes

The various stages of thought and reasoning suggest a growth in capability of processing information, increasing with age and maturity. Is this suggestion correct? Can we observe special features in human thinking? Let us take a look at what experimental psychology has discovered. We shall base the following ideas mainly on the studies of Miller (1956a, b) and Mandler (1967a, b).

In respect of thought processes the brain can be thought of as having two compartments: the compartment of short term memory (STM) and that of long term memory (LTM), terms which were introduced by James (1890). It is widely held that the characteristics of information processing are:

(1) it operates essentially serially, one process at a time;

(2) the inputs and outputs of these processes are held in a small STM with the capacity of only a few symbols;

(3) the system has access to an essentially infinite LTM, which has a fast retrieval rate, but a slow storage (Simon and Newell, 1970).

The bottleneck of the system seems to be the STM because of its severe limitation in processing capacity. In his entertaining and illuminating paper Miller (1956) proposed an ingenious model which can explain many of the questions raised in trying to understand human information processing. Miller suggests that the limiting value for information processing in STM is the 'magical number seven, plus or minus two'. Miller calls this value the channel capacity which can be defined as 'the upper limit on the extent to which an observer can match his responses to the stimuli that are given to him.'

People usually cannot distinguish more than about seven alternatives of a uni-dimensional variable, nor can they remember more than about seven items from an input list in immediate memory. Given these limitations, some mechanism must be responsible for extending human judgement and memory, since we obviously do remember more than seven items and can judge across a wider range. Miller's solution to this puzzle was, in the case of human memory, the unitization hypothesis.

The unitization hypothesis states, first, that the memory limit cannot be extended by simply adding more sets of seven items because the second set of seven apparently makes us forget the first. We are all aware of this aspect; when our wives asks us to attend to some errand, we are likely to forget the errand when we have other things on our mind. The only way to extend the amount of information is to enrich each item, i.e., to increase the amount of information each item conveys (Mandler, 1967). An enriched item is referred to as a 'chunk'. A 'chunk' is defined as 'any structure that has become familiar from previous repeated exposure and hence is recognizable as a single unit'. Whereas the 'chunk' is an enriched item, a single item is called a 'bit'. One bit of information is the amount of information we need to make a decision between two equally likely alternatives. So, 1 bit distinguishes 2 alternatives, 2 bits 4 alternatives, 3 bits 8, etc. The general rule becomes simple: every time the number of alternatives is increased by a factor two, one bit of information is added. Essentially, the STM is limited by the number of items which can be either bits or also chunks.

'By organizing the stimulus input simultaneously into several dimensions and successively into a sequence of chunks, we manage to break the informational bottleneck'. (There is a great deal of evidence to suggest that experts in any field think in terms of chunks whilst the novice regards the same information in smaller units.) In the language of communication theory this process is called recoding. The input is given in a code that contains many chunks with few bits per chunk. The problem-solver recodes the input into another code that contains fewer chunks with more bits per chunk. There are many ways to do this recoding, but probably the simplest one is to group the input events, apply a new name to the group, and then remember the new name rather than the original events' (Miller).

Recoding is an extremely powerful weapon for increasing the amount of information we can deal with. In one form or another, we use recoding constantly in our daily behaviour. When we want to remember we rephrase it 'in our own words': we make a verbal description of the event and then remember our own verbalization (compare this with the defining of abstract (medical) names to aggregates of symptoms and signs: Chapter I).

Drawings or pictures are more rapidly categorized than words, i.e., drawings lead to more rapid judgements as to whether what is presented does or does not belong to a particular category. People can therefore access conceptual information about the objects directly from pictures without having to name the object, even implicitly. This implies that category information is not tied to a verbal system, but instead can be accessed non-verbally. Information is represented abstractly and removed from the sensory systems that give rise to it (Squibb, 1987). Physicians often remember particular symptom-patterns from a specific patient case. This patient case represents the standard to which new patients will be compared. The specific elements within this symptom-pattern often have a more abstract meaning as they are stripped from their original sensory modality.

Is there an upper limit to the amount of information in a chunk? According to Mandler the limiting value for bits per chunk is again about $7^{+}/_{-}2$. This does not imply that memory is limited to 49 items. The process goes on to a next level of organization, where the first order chunks are recoded in 'super-chunks' with the same limit applying to this level, and so forth. In the organization of words as items chunking proceeds as a process of categorization of words eventually leading to a hierarchical system of subcategories, categories and supercategories. It may be clear that this process of chunking or categorizing is a very personal affair as it is mainly based on experience. Not only is the way of chunking or categorizing very personal, so is the combination of categories, the hierarchical structuring of categories, and the recoding or renaming.

Each individual carries his own idiosyncratic system of chunks. Chunks are expressions of personal experience. The experience of each individual determines more or less the ease or the difficulty of the information processing. Items of information with a high taxonomic frequency have significantly greater recall and chunking values than those of low taxonomic frequency. In other words, taxonomic frequency is one variable that affects the likelihood that a category will be discovered and used. The same is true for highly overlearned categories. Every doctor sharply recalls the symptoms and signs of the diseases of the acute abdomen, as he is taught over and over again that the consequences of missing them is disastrous to the patient as well as to the doctor.

The process of memory storage and recall

Another interesting finding is that subjective organization (recoding by the individual) leads to better recall and chunking than imposed organization (recoding suggested by teachers, etc.) Indeed, imposed organization even interferes with the efficiency of recall and chunking.

Recall can be impaired by various mechanisms.

(1) As we all know our concentration for recall can be seriously diverted by means of several interfering circumstances. A sudden noise can break our line of thought, flashes of light, even if they are observed from the corner of the eye, may disturb the concentration, etc. Generally, visual representations are more seriously impaired by visual interferences and auditory by auditory interferences, etc. Interference is more or less tied to the modality from which the representation originates. The effect of interference is reduced by pausing.

(2) Deficient recognition. In order to observe analogy we must have the ability to recognize as well as the potential to appreciate the meaning of

the familiar material. In brain dysfunction these capabilities can diminish and even disappear. In cases of dementia (e.g., Alzheimer's disease) people often do not recognize familiar faces or situations, and when they recognize them they do not grasp the meaning. For instance, the patient does not recognize his grandchildren, and when recognized he places them in a complete different context (different parents, different towns, etc.).

Memory abilities depend on highly developed skills for recoding, encoding and organisation of a particular piece of information. By properly organising specific pieces of information into a particular category the processing of data as well as the ability to remember these data can be markedly enhanced. However, the number of items which can be remembered from a category is limited. The number of items people remembered from a category was found to be 5.6 on average, while recall was a direct function of the number of categories used. In a less specified experiment and with small numbers of categories we found a figure of 4.5 on average. Mandler found that with a small number of categories individuals have a greater tendency (a) to switch from category to category during recall, or (b) to use categories not evaluated by the categorizing task. We found in our study a rather disperse distribution of the categories.

In his famous experiments de Groot (1946, 1965) confronted experienced chess players with specific groupings of pieces. Allowing only a quick glance at an authentic game position he asked chess players of various gradation (grandmasters, class players, beginners) to replace the groupings of the pieces on an empty chess board. The most experienced chess players remembered the perceived groupings very well (16 correctly placed pieces out of 26) in contrast with beginners (4 out of 26). The grandmasters could easily replace the pieces because of previously remembered game positions (they remembered 'grouping-chunks'), whereas the beginners had only a scattered picture of the game position. When the pieces were randomly distributed on the board and the same instruction was given, the ability levels disappeared.

Apparently, subjective organisation plays a relatively important role in memory storage and recall. However, when the organisation is imposed upon the pupil (for instance, recoding suggested by teachers) the effects of memory recall were less conspicuous. Imposed organisation will even interfere with the efficiency of recall and chunking.

Another phenomenon with regard to information organisation deserves attention. Lichtenstein *et al.* (1978) found that people tend to organise observed events in 'masses', as opposed to dispersed in time. In their opinion occurrences have a tendency to manifest themselves in outcrops. 'Massing of data' enables people to economize their information processing, but, on the other hand, also influences people's estimation of occurrences. In the judges' opinion, occurrences tend to be massed rather than distributed over time. For example, people believe air crashes to occur in series, physicians believe myocardial infarction to happen in outbreaks.

The 'massing of data' may be an explanation for differences between laboratory and real life experiments, the former mainly derived of sensational or emotional charges or items. People respond heavily to emotionally charged events, especially when stressed to be catastrophic. They exhibit strong and often consistent biases. Some portion of these errors may be due to the unrepresentative coverage of these events in news media. Zebrowski (quoted in Lichtenstein *et al.*) notes that 'fear sells': media dwell on potential catastrophes and not on successful operations. The more that is published about some kind of disease, the more the physician tends to diagnose it. Not only the physician but the patient also is influenced by this psychological effect. It effects the presentation of the complaint. Lichtenstein *et al.* found two explanations:

   (a) encoding variability: spaced repetitions are more likely to receive differential coding than massed items;
   (b) deficient processing of massed items. The studies of Tversky and Kahnemann (1974) made clear that people tend to estimate weights of events and their frequency by a number of erroneous heuristics. As estimates play an essential role in medical decision-making, this matter will be discussed in Chapter IV.

The process of forgetting

Apart from these limitations, there is another restriction imposed on information processing and memory storage and recall: the loss of memory, the tendency to forget. We shall illustrate this by the study of Bower (1967). In Bower's model information is labelled by a code (encoding) and stored as a compound vector. Assuming that a compound vector CB is stored as a vector of information components forgetting would consist in the blurring, erasure, or change in value of some of the components of the initial vector. As forgetting proceeds and the trace (= CB) is further degraded, it conveys less and less information about the initiating event B. The vector will usually consist of many components, some or all of which may function as a recall trigger. If the value of a given component of the trace has been erased, the recall function is obliterated.

Events that are encoded similarly, with few distinguishing features, will be readily confused in recall. The range of confusion errors in recall will increase with the number of the forgotten components. It would be said that the individual retains the general gist of the events for some time but that he becomes more and more vague or inaccurate about the exact details. Bower suggests two theoretical hypotheses in the process of forgetting.

   (I)   The components are forgotten in a strict hierarchical order, from most detailed to most general information, and the last component being forgotten first, then the next, and so on; or they are forgotten independently regardless of their possible location in a hierarchy of importance.
   (II) A forgotten value of a component is replaced by a null state or is replaced by some other value selected at random.

With regard to the former hypothesis, there is no evidence for the thought of hierarchical ordering. So the probability of a correct recall is a function only of the number of bits forgotten and is independent of their location in the hierarchical sorting tree.

With regard to the second hypothesis two theories exist. According to one view the forgotten component is reverted to a null state. On recall, when a null state is encountered, the recall function chooses at random (guesses) among the values at the position in constructing or locating a response. According to the alternate view the value is replaced by a non-null value. Here the recall function reacts as if there is a real value; it is tricked by its memory into believing that all components are known. In our study we found that most doctors have some kind of absolute belief in their memory recall, not only mirroring the real state(s) but being complete also. Kochen (1983), however, found that physicians remembered cases and what exactly was done in only 5%. This figure differs sharply from what doctors themselves think to be their best knowledge base, experience. In the study of Kochen he found that physicians rely for their decisions mostly on their experience and only for 24% on the knowledge gathered in the medical school.

It may be clear that the 'null-state' hypothesis leads to 'fuzzy' memories regarded by the person with low confidence as to their accuracy. The second, the non-null-state, hypothesis will lead to clear but inaccurate memories. It is these latter memories that trouble most.

Mandler (1967) reports a sharp initial decay of memory but no further loss, even after three or four months. Using a single word as trigger for a category or vector, recall drops from 90% to about 75% in the first six weeks and stabilizes at approximately 50%–60% after the seventh week. The immediate recall for a category is 98%.

A subsequent dilemma is the fate of partly forgotten memory vectors, remnants of categories. It is suggested that residues of categories, especially those in which initial components are encoded similarly and with few distinguishing features, are combined in order to form a 'new' category. The clustering of the remnants, as an efficient act for organizing the memory, takes place unconsciously. We become aware of these new categories in our dreams, when parts of various situations, referring to different categories, come into our half-consciousness. However, it may be possible that several notions, opinions, remembrances, etc., really come into the consciousness with a strong belief in the truthfulness of this recall. Witnesses can fervently adhere to a particular judgement or description although opposing evidence is available. They are convinced of the truthfulness of their testimony.

Especially in medicine where the memory search for 'similar' cases plays so strong a role, these memory tricks may fool the physician and it may often lead him, when not guided by reliable acquired evidence, in the wrong directions. On the other hand, the acquisition of evidence is limited by the channel capacity of the short term memory. There seem to be two ways to overcome this restriction. He can note down all the information at the moment of the interview or he can cluster the collected information into a 'meaningful' category or working hypothesis. The recording of all symptoms and signs during the interview or examination is rather unusual, as we have explained in Chapter I, 4. It strongly interferes with the doctor-patient communication and distracts the physician from his, more or less pre-planned, problem-solving process. Recording of the patient's evidence takes place mainly after the consultation, with, unfortunately, all the possibilities of a deficient memory recall. Although overtly encouraging the physician-participants in our investigation (see Chapter VI) to note down the presented information, it was, however, hardly practised. Only a few notes were made during the consultation.

The possibility of clustering the information into meaningful (for the doctor and for no one else) categories was demonstrated in all 253 patient cases as solved by 68 physicians. They moved from one category to another with, to our surprise, a rather fixed number of questions (to the patient) in between. When we define the move from one category to another as one cycle, we discovered the following result:

TABLE I

Cycle	Mean number of questions
1	17.20
2	16.64
3	15.46
4	15.47
5	17.44
6	18.67

These figures seem scarcely to sustain Miller's theory. However, we have to realize that on average the doctor returned to one of the symptoms twice during each interview. Besides, pair-wise questioning is commonly practised in doctor-patient interviews. Think of, for instance, tiredness and dizziness, or, nausea and vomiting, or, thirst and abundant urinating, dyspnea and nocturnal miction, etc., etc. We are unable to analyze this aspect from our material but we think that this table is, nevertheless, suggestive of the channel capacity restrictions of the thought processes as they were predicted by Miller.

The problem of forgetting is especially apposite to clinical practice. We found that physicians frequently reason by analogy. For that reason he scans his memory for similar cases, or supposedly similar cases. When he cannot find a satisfying similarity he often makes a wild guess, a diagnosis out of the blue. Supposed similarity also often came from cases he had recently encountered in practice. Although the similarity was based on a superficial resemblance, he, nevertheless, stuck to his idea even if the presented evidence strongly suggested otherwise.

It is the problem of the presumed similarity, the superficial resemblance, the mistaken analogy that can lead doctors into erroneous thinking and conclusions. As the similarity, the analogy, is based on (deficient) memory, on inexact recall, or on combinations of memory remnants, and on individual chunking, this type of reasoning is unsuited for intra-disciplinary or inter-disciplinary audit.

Problem-solving in complex tasks

Faced with a problem-solving task of challenging complexity, an individual may try to restructure that task into a simpler one. This can be accomplished in two ways: scanning his memory for similar and known cases, or by combining data in known categories.

I. Restructure of the problem

The problem is dismantled to its bare bones and the number of alternatives is limited. The larger the number of alternatives and their consequences which have to be assessed, the poorer the quality of a person's thinking will be. The person therefore preferentially brings the complex, multi-dimensional task back to a uni-dimensional one. In daily life people tend to think in simple cause-consequence patterns, although most situations are far more complex. Reasoning like, 'criminality is caused by unemployment', or 'the threat of war is caused by the arms race', etc., is rather common in the media. A very complicated disease of which hypertension is only a symptom is reduced to observing the elevated blood pressure. When elderly people become mentally confused the problem is often reduced to the diagnosis of dementia without much consideration of alternative explanations.

II. Limiting the information

(a) People try to avoid (or disregard) data which can possibly lead to negative outcomes (Balla, 1980). People tend to focus on the number of true positives while following the strategy of using only confirming evidence (Brehmer, 1980).

(b) The limitation of the data can also be accomplished by the restriction of the search procedure to combinations of informational elements, e.g., correlated symptoms, preferably those symptoms that either have both typical or both atypical characteristics (Medin et al., 1982). People tend to look for correlations even if the information contained in the correlation is less than each of the parts. These correlations can consist of a combination of two symptoms as well as complete symptom-patterns. Evidently the sum of the correlated symptoms counts higher than the summation of each of them separately. Correlations of single or complex symptoms are presumably based on experience and personal knowledge.

Studies of physicians' thought processes

Our first and fundamental question was: 'do recognisable strategies exist according to which a (family) physician arrives at a decision?' Several authors deny the existence of anything like a particular or recognisable strategy or strategies. It is claimed that, because of the uniqueness of the patient-physician relation, every physician has not only his particular way of working, but he also has manifold strategies at his disposal, for each problem a different strategy. But the remarkable phenomenon exists that physicians all over the world, providing they are using 'Western Medicine', recognize each other's methods, schemes and problems. It reaches beyond the borders set by cultures, societies or health care systems. What is this peculiar thing that connects physicians all over the world?. .What is the characteristic (are the characteristics) that makes physicians recognisable to each other?

Of course, one of the elements is the patient presenting his problem. But this cannot explain everything. We suggest that a joint strategy(or strategies) is a major element in connecting physicians all over the world. Literature on this subject is scarce. The first signs of interest can be traced back to the 'fifties, when investigators, mainly working for departments of education, tried to restructure medical examinations. Rimoldi (1955) tried to simulate the medical process by means of written information and instruction.

During the 'sixties several instruments like *Patient Management Problem* (McGuire, 1967), *Diagnostic Management Problem* (Helfer and Slater, 1970), P_4 (Tamblyn and Barrows, 1978) etc., tried to simulate the problem-solving and thought processes of expert clinicians in order to study their thought processes and at the same time to use these instruments to educate and examine the medical students. They were all basically normative as they implicitly used a model of assumed clinical reasoning as it was explained to the experimenters by expert clinicians. As we mentioned, we agree with Sober (1979) that 'the clinician's description of his clinical diagnosis is no more than a rationalization. It is false to the facts of his own psychological processes'. Put to trial these models failed to predict the accuracy of the problem-solving processes of experienced physicians (Newble and Hoare, 1982). Evidently, they do not mimic the physicians' thought processes.

Another model was developed by Ledley, a mathematician, and Lusted, a radiologist. Their interesting and intriguing paper 'Reasoning foundations of medical diagnosis' (1959) is still viewed as the starting-point of clinical decision analysis. They analyzed the medical process as they had conceptualized it. They structured it into a logical and probabilistic system. They introduced decision theory (borrowed from economic science) into the medical discipline which enabled them to calculate predictive values for particular symptoms and diagnoses. It soon became clear that the medical process, as these authors had conceptualised, only represented a theoretical basis which could serve as a model for further developments in the world of clinical decision-making. It did not simulate the actual process in routine clinical practice.

Next to this, two other methods were developed, both originating in cognitive psychology. In a non-chronological order they can be described as

(1) multiple branching method, and
(2) artificial intelligence.

The first goes back to the Gestalt[1] psychologists, Duncker (on problem-solving) and Wertheimer (*Productive Thinking*, 1945). The theory of concept formation was further developed and led to experiments with psychologists (Mandler, 1967; Kleinmuntz, 1968) and clinicians (Wortman, 1972, 1971). The latter author tested Mandler's theory about the organization of information in memory into hierarchical structures. Wortman found three stages of a recoding process: (a) the perception of the hierarchy of categories; (b) chunking within a subordinate category; and (c) the establishment of the hierarchical relationship between superordinate and subordinate categories. This led to a multiple branching scheme of organizational hierarchy.

Multiple branching can be seen as a logical progression down one of the many possible paths in which the response to each test or question automatically determines the next step. This scheme is more widely known as a decision tree giving each step the weight of a probability estimation towards a previously determined outcome (see Chapter IV).

Wortman's model was based on a 'thinking aloud' procedure of a neurologist. We suppose that the rationalization of the clinical process, the model in mind, and the 'thinking aloud' method all contributed to a schema that hardly seems to resemble the thought processes of a practising physician.

Artificial intelligence, although it seems a brand new branch of science, goes back to the beginning of this century. The experiments of Wundt gave a fresh impulse to epistemology. Especially the philosophical theories of Selz (*'Ueber die Gesetze des Geordneten Denkverlaufs'*[2] (1913); *'Die Gesetze der Produktiven und Reproduktiven Geistestaetigkeit'*[3] (1924)), influenced investigators to more practical theories such as cybernetics (Norbert Wiener, 1948). Cybernetics was a general name encompassing three systems:

(1) information theory;
(2) theory of feedback systems (servomechanism theory); and
(3) the system of electronic computing. When we know what is going on in the human mind, we must be able to simulate the process.

The advantage of the information processing approach is its possibility to retrace the various steps in the process. As the problem-solving activities are supposed to be directed by the problem, the problem-solving space reflects the organizational structure of memory in information processing as well as in human problem-solving. In other words, an information processing approach can simulate human behaviour problem-solving. It will lead to the formulation of a number of conditions for a problem-solving programme or simulation.

Several programmes based on the 'thought' models of artificial intelligence have been designed. Most of these programmes are presently known as 'expert system' as they ought to mimic the reasoning processes of experts. Inherent to the construction of these systems are the conditions formulated by Simon and Newell in 1971:

[1] Gestalt: German for: figure, form, shape.
[2] About the laws of regulated thinking processes.
[3] The laws of productive and reproductive mental activities.

(1) it should predict the performance of a problem-solver handling specific tasks;
(2) it should explain how human problem-solving takes place;
(3) what processes are used;
(4) what mechanisms perform these processes;
(5) it should predict the incidental phenomena that accompany the problem-solving process.

These conditions are not always met in simulations and investigations in medical informatics. In our opinion this omission alienated the physicians from this formalized approach in medical decision-making. The information processing programmes became less and less recognisable to the practising physician, which resulted in disillusion and lack of interest. On the other hand, information scientists became annoyed by the physician's behaviour. Their straightforward and clear (in their opinion) programmes and algorithms had not been accepted by the physicians; indeed, they were rejected.

In our opinion, three obstacles towards amalgamation of the formalized and the 'informal' ways of problem-solving and decision-making can be distinguished:
(1) the 'reasoning' strategies of the formalized and those of the practising physician differ too much;
(2) physicians know, or at least intuitively feel, that the variability and unreliability of the medical data makes accurate calculation of the various probabilities (when at all possible) nearly impossible (and therefore cannot be relied upon);
(3) the formalized systems have been mainly restricted to very narrowly circumscribed areas of medical practice. They are of little interest to the practising physician.

The validity of inference

People commonly view their memories as exact copies of their original experiences. During reconstruction, a variety of cognitive, social and motivational factors can introduce error and distortion into the output from memory recall.

If one is unaware of the reconstructive nature of memory and perception, one cannot distinguish between assertion and inferences; one will not critically evaluate one's inferred knowledge. In general, any process that changes the contents of memory unbeknownst to people will keep them from asking relevant validity questions and may lead to overconfidence (Fischhoff *et al.*, 1977). Wason and Johnson-Laird (1972) have shown subjects having considerable confidence in their own erroneous reasoning. The inferences had not been arrived at as a series of logical steps but swiftly and almost unconsciously.

The validity of the inference was usually not inquired into; indeed, the process was usually accompanied by a feeling of certainty of being right (Fischhoff *et al.*). The strategies of the inference processes seem to differ from subject to subject. The subject's strategy becomes a crucial intervening variable between the task environment in which he works and the behaviour he produces. Some strategies may be more effective than others, but effective strategies may be difficult to discover. It is hardly likely, particularly in unfamiliar tasks, that all subjects will come equipped with the best strategies or will be able to find them during the problem-solving setting. Subjects tend to use various kinds of heuristics to restrict their domain. The selectivity of search (confirmation) and the urge for speed, is taken as a key organizing principle. There is a strong tendency to confirm the hypothesis directly. The strategy of disconfirming alternatives is less automatic.

When the rules fail, they tend to assume that there is no rule at all. They use some sort of memorization strategy or they give up and guess (Brehmer, 1980). Wason and Johnson-Laird (1972) wonder why subjects fail to follow adequate logical rules. They suggest that subjects do not understand the logical relation of implication ('if', 'then') but tend to consider this relation equivalent to a double implication 'if, and only if'. Hypotheses were not properly tested although the optimal rule to help them was given.

It was assumed that subjects will employ deductive inferences with an eye on logic; instead they use various and varying heuristic rules according to time, environment and personality. The reason may be that they lack the necessary basic schemata to help them understand and use the information provided by their experiences. Subjects have the intuitive understanding that non-randomness is information, and information can be exploited to search a problem space in promising directions and to avoid the less promising. A little information goes a long way to keep within bounds the amount of search required, on average, to find the solution (Simon and Newell, 1971).

When they encounter some symptom ordering or patterns, or a memorized correlation, subjects feel at ease. It will direct their pathway through the problem space. This is especially interesting when conclusions or patterns are formulated early in the process. However, they can be misleading and may direct attention to irrelevant features of the problem, cause the subject to engage in a search for inconsequential cues that would otherwise be ignored, or lead the decision-maker to refrain from useful search for cues that would otherwise be collected. But it certainly helps the physicians in their daily practice as it provides speed and the feeling of sensible working on a problem.

What is a problem?

The English Platonist Weldon said that there are three kinds of element that people are concerned about regarding the thinking processes of man. There are troubles which we do not quite know how to handle; there are puzzles whose conditions and unique solutions are quite clear to everybody; and there are problems. We invent a problem by finding an appropriate puzzle form to impose upon a trouble.

Before a person can attempt to solve a problem, he must understand or assimilate a description of the problem. The presentation of a trouble or a complaint does not automatically imply the understanding by the problem-solver. There are at least two conditions to this understanding;

(a) it can be a problem only if it puzzles or worries somebody (assimilation) (Polanyi, 1968); and

(b) a translation of the problem can be made in such a way that it becomes a familiar type of problem to the problem-solver, for which he has means within his repertoire for solving it (acquisition) (Mettes, 1980).

The first condition refers to the situation that something is called a problem when it pertains to a task for which the respective subject does not immediately perceive a way of finding a solution. It means that every problem has its individual and personal character. This is reflected in the definition of Thorndike (1911):

> 'A problem exists when the goal that is sought is not directly attainable by the performance of a simple act available in the personal repertory; the solution calls for either a novel action or a new integration of available action'.

Most people prefer to avoid problems, especially the complicated ones. Politicians confronted with complex, multi-faceted dilemmas will try to satisfy their constituents, rather than struggle with basic solutions to the dilemmas. Judges asked to settle a major legal controversy will often make their decision not by directly resolving the substantial issue, but by evading it, reaching a conclusion based on matters of technical procedure. Facing a problem means facing the highly personal dilemma of making decisions. And people are constantly being reminded of what they already know from personal experience – that making a consequential decision is a worrisome thing, and one is liable to lose sleep over it. We cannot but recognize and smile at the cartoonist's statement in Peanuts: 'No problem is too big or too complicated that it cannot be run away from!' (cited in Janis and Mann, 1977).

Evidently, the problem solver needs stimulation and motivation to tackle a problem and to proceed in order to find a solution. To this end a number of conditions have to be fulfilled.

- Interest in a case. Our interest in a case is raised by the pre-known, the various experiences which determine the relevance we shall apply to the case at hand.

- Familiarity. The last thing anyone would be likely to solve is an unfamiliar problem. When a problem cannot be fitted into our conceptual viewpoint and task-environment, it is very unlikely that a solution will emerge (except for some moral standpoint).

- Foreknowledge. To be accepted as a problem the question must be recognised as such. 'Doctor, when I blink with my right eye it hurts in my left foot' is not recognised by the physician as a real problem. Obviously, the question posed must fit into his discipline, his attention, and his field of experience.

- Acceptance of the solution. When a person has the strong feeling that any solution whatsoever to a problem will not be accepted, he will feel less inclined to proceed with problem-solving. When a patient refuses in advance some particular treatment, e.g., surgery, the physician will no

longer search for a solution but will only scan his memory for some alternative treatment, perhaps less appropriate.
- Time limits. The problem solver must at least have the impression that he is able to find a solution within a given time span. When he assumes the time span to be inadequate, he will tend to rely on less optimal decision-making; in the extreme case this lead to panic (see, e.g., Janis and Mann, 1977: *Emergency Decision-making*). In clinical emergency cases physicians do not solve the problem but take a number of actions to create and ensure a time span in which they possibly can find a solution.

Most of these elements are usually completely obscure. The individual has no idea which factors influence the process. Sometimes even the fact that the process is taking place is unknown to the individual prior to the point that a solution appears in his consciousness.

What is a medical problem?

Patients do not present 'problems' to the doctor: they present a number of complaints or signs which they observe as deviant from their normal pattern of physical, psychical and/or social functioning. From these features they present only a small part: the part they think to be relevant to the physician. They present the signs according to their understanding of the medical world and medical problem-solving, their notion of 'normality' and 'normal functioning'. But what we do not know is how complete a portion of the total picture of signs and symptoms the patient reveals.

Obviously, the patient presents his unresolved problem to the physician as someone whom he believes to be a more competent and professional problem solver. It is up to the physician to understand what the patient's problem is. Boshuizen and Claessen (1982) raise the interesting question whether the physician solves the patient's problem or is occupied with his own diagnostic task. The answer is that each has his own personal agenda.

As we have argued previously, a problem can only be perceived as a problem when it is assimilated into a personal puzzle, which then needs translation into a familiar context in order to catch and solve it. This does not imply that the physician immediately perceives a way towards finding a solution, but he recognizes it as belonging to his task environment.

The patient-physician contact can be sketched as follows.

(1) A person experiences some troubles which become a problem by some kind of social process. Parsons (1951) found that some kind of acknowledgement is required before an individual can enter the 'sick role'. His or her perception of disturbed health needs a sort of approval from the family, job partners, and other social relations. Patients entering the 'sick role' have their own concepts of disease. Because the 'sick role' provides a person with certain privileges, this concept is not free from personal values. The doctor's role is to define illness, confer the sick status on potential patients, establish priorities, and take the initiative in evaluating health status and controlling health problems (Brody, 1980).

Redlich (1976) describes two stages, referred to as sick role I and II. The patient in sick role I assumes that

(a) he is not responsible for these changes (they are not voluntary and not punishable);

(b) he is excused from his ordinary social and occupational obligations; and

(c) he is expected to strive to get well as expediently as possible.

Acknowledged as a 'patient' by the physician, he enters sick role II, in which it is assumed that

(1) he will drop or modify his own system of thinking; and

(2) adopt the physician's system, especially if clear professional information is offered to him.

This not only puts the responsibility in the hands of the physician, but it may also lead clinicians to confuse symptoms with socio-cultural patterns of behaviour associated with help-seeking.

(2) Based on the patient's appreciation of his problem and his expectation about the medical competence, he may turn to the medical care institution(s) or the physician.

(3) The patient presents (pieces of) his unresolved problem to the physician expecting to receive some advice or prescription for some course of action which will enable him to solve his problem. However, this ideally typified procedure hardly ever takes place. According to Redlich (1976) the patient is expected to adopt the physician's system. The implications of this behaviour may determine – to a great extent – the attitudes of the participants towards the processes of illness and treatment and to the health experience.

(4) From the presented data the physician creates his own problem. This means that every medical problem has its own personal character. A medical problem, therefore, is the highly individualistic translation (by the physician) of a highly individualistic presentation (by the patient) of a complaint.

(5) The physician solves the perception of the problem as presented by the patient. We must be aware that great differences may exist between the patient's problem and the perceived one; they do not always happen to coincide. As mentioned previously, the message must yield some medical significance. However, the conceptions of medical significance of the doctor and of the patient can differ widely.

(6) The solution at which the doctor arrives must be communicated to the patient and, moreover, be accepted by him. We cannot accept the idea that the patient's mind is a clean slate upon which the doctor engraves his prescription. The patient has, consciously or unconsciously, formed an idea about possible solutions. They might be horrifying or reassuring, acceptable or unacceptable, but patients have their own problem-solving system. Adaption of the problem-solving-system of the doctor to that of the patient's is a necessary condition for the solution of the patient's problem.

We can sketch this situation in the following schema.

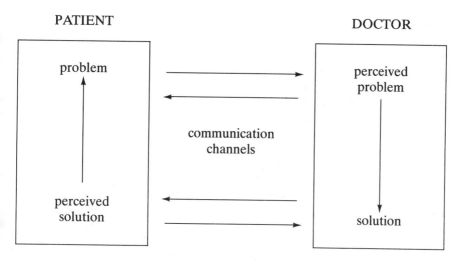

(7) The patient has to connect the offered/perceived solution to his original
     problem. The extensive literature on non-compliance is an illustration
     of the fact that this connection does not always take place. It leaves the
     patient in a rather difficult position. He has committed himself to an
     expert who asks him to accept the offered solution. But where the
     patient cannot accept the solution as satisfactory, he has to reconsider
     his position with regard to the doctor in whom he confides. Only a small
     number of alternatives are left to the patient. One of them is an
     alternative doctor.

A medical problem cannot be regarded as an element that can be standardized and categorized. Attempts to categorize and classify medical problems
seem questionable. Different perceptions of health disturbance, different
abilities in coping, different social and professional backgrounds, different
education, different social levels (to the physician), different culture and
language, and different appreciation of the health care system, are all factors
creating thresholds in the appreciation of the patient's troubles. The question
of who is healthy and who is not is a matter of great inherent ambiguity that is
actively negotiated between those people with complaints and other people
ranging from members of the immediate family, friends and neighbours to
people presumed to know about health matters because of personal experiences, special training, or connections with the medical care system (Twaddle,
1982).

Not only does the presentation of the illness vary, the illness behaviour also
influences the physician's identification of the problem (Korsch and Negrete,
1974; Mechanic, 1972; Zola, 1963). The patient's behaviour can direct the
physician's attention to certain features while he neglects others. For example,

a physical presentation can distract the physician from psychical or social aspects of the presented illness and vice versa.

Another disturbing factor can be the way in which patients and physicians communicate. 'Talking to people is a doctor's game that doctors don't play'. This overstatement illustrates the kind of difficulties which may arise in patient-physician contact. The extensive literature on patient-physician communication examplifies this particular issue.

'Doctors observe little and they observe badly', as Lasegue noted more than a century ago. This rather cynical statement raises the question of the precise and accurate observation, by the physician, of the symptoms and signs in the patient, in order to know what the medical problem is. Some studies (Cochrane *et al.*, 1951, Koran, 1975a, 1975b) about inter-observer (recordings of clinical observations between various physicians) and intra-observer (recording of observations of one physician over periods of time) variabilities underscore the difficulties physicians face in observing the patient's symptoms and signs. Wulff (1976) noted the impossibility of applying precise measures to the questioning and examining procedure since the patient cannot be questioned several times about the same symptom without one answer affecting the others. However, the truth (accuracy) of the patient's answers must usually be taken for granted.

The health problems presented by the patient represent abstractions of disease manifestations. They are largely generalisations based on experience, and it is not expected that all (or even most) patients with a given disease will present signs and symptoms which exactly match the predefined pattern.

Nevertheless, the chief complaint, its allied symptoms, related physical signs and laboratory and X-ray information must be grouped into a category, a diagnosis, a name of a disease. Having classified the disease the physician is able to outline a course of action and treatment.

Problem space and task environment

Before a person can attempt to solve a problem it needs translation into a familiar type of problem in order to lead him to the next phase of searching for a solution. Unfamiliar problems are beyond the reach of our skills. Physicians need plumbers to solve their leakage problems, plumbers need mechanics to fix their car problems, and mechanics need doctors to solve their ailments. In order to be able to attack a problem the problem solver defines a problem space. A problem space consists mainly of states of knowledge about the problem and rules relevant to the various states; for instance, a mathematical problem can be solved by the application of the relevant know-how and the pertinent rules. The problem space for the doctor can be described as his particular medical knowledge relevant to the case and the particular way of reasoning in order to solve this clinical problem.

As the physician's medical knowledge is partly experiential knowledge and the rules of problem-solving more or less idiosyncratic ones, the problem space also includes the prejudices and prejudgements of the doctor. Chapman and

Chapman (1967) demonstrated how prior expectations can lead to erroneous observations and inferences. People tend to see what they want and expect to see because of their 'foreknowledge' of a case. This can lead to a number of implications, among which are:

- it more or less directs the problem-solving. Medin *et al.* (1982) saw more pattern-recognition when there was an assumed resemblance to cases presented a short time before;
- it largely conceals the details of the process;
- it inhibits an evaluation of the judgement processes by preventing a careful consideration of the various options;
- it introduces bias into guesswork.

In family medicine, where physicians are proud of their foreknowledge of the patient these implications pose a serious risk.

Most of these elements are usually completely obscure. The individual has no idea which factor influence the process. Sometimes even the fact that the process is taking place is unknown to the individual prior to the point that a solution appears in his consciousness.

Sometimes the problem is translated and transformed to a task the problem solver thinks he is capable of tackling. This means, for instance, that the physician translates the patient's problem into a task he can understand within the context of medical science and health care. For example, many doctors, especially family physicians, are often confronted with problems beyond their special competence like problems of a social, educational or psychological nature. Frequently they try to relate these problems to domains in which they feel more confident, e.g., a clinical domain. The reverse can also be observed: the doctor who attributes clinical problems to elements of stress, matrimonial disharmony, etc. Thus can the doctor be led astray even at the very beginning of the problem-solving process.

It is the task environment which determines the physician's problem space and its boundaries, because, being a doctor, he is only partly responsible for creating the task environment. Social, cultural, administrative, and professional influences effect the climate, the task environment of the single physician. The physician is bound to offer his services by virtue of his Hippocratic oath; he has to treat patients irrespective of their nature, colour, or behaviour; he is obliged to act because even non-acting is his responsibility.

This means that the task (and its environment) mainly determines the characteristics of the problem-solving process (Newell and Simon, 1972). Simon and Newell (1971) summarize these characteristics as follows:

(1) a few, and only a few, gross characteristics of the human information processing system are invariable over the task and problem solver;
(2) these characteristics are sufficient to determine that a task environment is represented as a problem space and that problem-solving takes place within the problem space;
(3) the structure of the task environment determines the possible structure;
(4) the structure of the problem space determines the possible programmes that can be used for the problem-solving.

Eventually this will lead to the formulation of a number of conditions for a problem-solving programme or simulation:

(a) it should predict the performance of a problem solver handling specific tasks;
(b) it should explain how human problem-solving takes place;
(c) what processes are used;
(d) what mechanisms perform these processes;
(e) it should predict the incidental phenomena that accompany the problem-solving process.

Problem-solving processes

'In medico-legal practice', Thorndyke remarked, 'one must be constantly on one's guard against the effects of suggestion, whether intentional or unconscious. When the facts of a case are set forth by an informant they are nearly always presented, consciously or unconsciously, in terms of inference. Certain facts, which appear to the narrator to be the leading facts, are given with emphasis and in detail, while other facts, which appear to be subordinate or trivial, are partially suppressed. But this assessment of evidential value must never be accepted. The whole case must be considered and each fact weighed separately and then it will commonly happen the leading fact turns out to be the one that had been passed over as negligible' (R. Austin Freeman, *The Stolen Ingots*).

The physician-author Austin Freeman knew what he was talking about. He was quite right that accurate problem-solving processes can be enhanced by following the advice to take the whole case into account. However, this approach, as used in his sparkling detective stories, is not always practical for the day-to-day medical practice. Physicians often have to adapt their problem-solving processes to the workload, which certainly detracts from optimal decision-making but gives them opportunities to survive. This survival process is something doctors are really proud of, and is often referred to as 'practice-experience' or 'good education of the patients'. They have learned in the end to cope with all the tricks and traps of routine clinical practice.

We are interested in what processes people and, more specifically, physicians *do* use to solve problems.

Animal studies led to the belief that problems are solved by trial and error. This concept led to a preference for observation instead of introspection. However, as Bertrand Russell (1927) remarked, animals tended to display the national characteristics of the experimenters: animals studied by Americans rush about frantically with an incredible display of hustle and pep, and at last achieve the desired result by chance. Animals observed by Germans sit still and think, and at last evolve the solution out of their inner consciousness (cited in Johnson-Laird and Wason, 1977).

But trial and error is, in fact, a rather limited and easy-going approach to problem-solving. In medicine this thought is rather unattractive, especially when it concerns ourselves. Although psychologists have generally studied the problem-solving processes from the viewpoint of deductive inference, tensions remain between these conscious deductions and everyday inferences. The inferences that underly deductive problem-solving are often slow, voluntary, and at the forefront of awareness: they are explicit. For practical reasons like alertness, quick reaction, workload, etc., this type of inference is scarcely used in routine problem-solving.

In contrast, the inferences that underlie the ordinary process of perception and comprehension are rapid, involuntary, and outside conscious awareness: they are implicit (Johnson-Laird and Wason, 1977).

The approach to problem-solving

Apart from trial and error two major schemes can be traced.
(1) Sequential: the solver always appears to search sequentially, adding small successive accretions to his store of information about the problem and its possible solution (Simon and Newell, 1971).
(2) Configural (Gestaltpsychology): the mind has 'the tendency to organize and integrate and to perceive situations, including problems, as total structures. The insight that leads to a solution, in the Gestalt view, stems from the perception of the requirements of a problem (Kohler, cited in Scheerer, 1963).

Both theories have in common the creation of a problem space which encompasses the elements of the problem, its related knowledge and rules and the – perception of a – solution. In Gestalt psychology the perception of the solution of a problem is like the perceiving of a hidden figure in a puzzle picture. That means that:
– the perception is sudden;
– there is no conscious intermediate stage;
– the relationships of the elements in the final perceptions are different from those which preceded them, i.e., changes in meaning are involved.
Translated to the medical situation it means that:
– a particular disease pattern in memory is called for;
– between the call and the 'jumping to the mind' no (logically) (re)traceable steps can be formulated nor observed;
– the disease pattern does not necessarily represent the exact replica of the memorized pattern: it shows a number of gross characteristics which mirror the original one.
The implications of this latter view are decisive. Because of its irreversible and irretraceable character the solution of the problem is perceived by the problem-solver as an actual discovery. But a discovery is only accredited as such when we believe that it comes from sheer induction, 'out of the blue' (Polanyi, 1958). But such a procedure hides the intermediate steps and makes the process irretraceable. While the sequential process can be made explicit by following the steps, the configurational one is unique, *'einmalig'*. This latter claim is often associated with the physician's problem-solving processes.

However, this does not mean that we now really understand cognitive processes. The bulk of the research on problem-solving has been carried out with naive subjects on tasks that do not call for much specific subject-matter knowledge, with scarcely any resemblance to real-life processes. The results of many experiments have given rise to pessimistic reactions. Recently, several cognitive psychologists (Mandler, 1975; Neisser, 1967; Miller, 1962) have proposed that we may have no direct access to higher order mental processes such as the ones involved in evaluation, judgement, problem-solving, and the imitation of behaviour.

Nisbett and Wilson (1977) agree with this statement arguing that verbal descriptions of recalled memories of problem-solving processes, (the so-called 'thinking-aloud' procedure), are 'telling more than you can know'. They argue that with or without stimulation any recall always carry traces of self-justification or some kind of theorizing. Ericsson and Simon (1980), however, maintain the possibility of verbal reports being reliable data for disclosing problem-solving processes as long as any recall that 'jumps to the mind' is noted down at the same instant as it is recalled.

New incentives have come from studies in Artificial Intelligence or the simulation of cognition, as Simon (1981) prefers to call it. Such simulation of cognition or creation of artificial intelligence contrasts with the modelling of the actual processes of human reasoning themselves. A system that simulates the reasoning of an expert clinician need only have similar input and output, but a system that models the reasoning process of an expert would also have to employ similar operations in generating the output from the input (Whitbeck and Brooks, 1983).

When trying to model a system on human cognition we must first learn how human cognition works. This is usually investigated by means of three types of model.

(A) Prescriptive models. On the basis of a (e.g., decision) theory a model is constructed which delineates and defines the process steps which have to be taken in order to reach an optimal outcome (e.g., an optimal decision). The model can act as a yardstick by which the performances of, e.g., the physicians can be measured.

(B) Descriptive models. The model tries to describe the context and factors which influence judgements. The descriptive model is largely concerned with the task environment of the problem solver. One of the most important descriptive models is the so-called 'lens' model of the American psychologist Brunswick (1952). He stressed the importance of studying not only a person's cognition but also the context in which the problem-solving processes take place.

(C) Process studies. Two types of studies can be identified. One type is exemplified by the Newell and Simon model (1972) which makes use of information science to construct a scheme which can simulate the problem solver's reasoning process. Another type is the process-tracing model. Process-tracing studies have mainly been carried out by subjects who reported in reflection their cognitive processes of preceding judgemental procedures. The validity of this type of study is seriously questioned because direct access to higher order mental processes is not open to either experimenter or subject. Hindsight reflection confuses the data (Nisbett and Wilson, 1977).

The existing models do not appeal to our ideas about the tracing of the physician's thought processes. Our aim was a 'real-life' process approach: an approach which could guide us by the observation of the patient-physician encounter in a real or simulated situation. However, real life studies often suffer from the bias of hindsight justification as they commonly make use of the so-called 'thinking aloud' procedure or 'stimulated recall' schema (interviewing the physician while he watches a video recorded tape of his own process).

In order to avoid the self-fulfilling prophecy of observing and infering what we wanted to observe or infer, a formal model of investigation is a necessary tool. This formal model has to reflect the problem-solving methods as they are used in 'real life', i.e., the routine clinical practice.

As we discussed above (Chapter II) we hypothesized the existence of two different methods as explanatory of the problem-solving and decision-making methods in clinical practice. The delineation and definition of these models will be described in Chapter V.

The number of investigations into these processes is rather small. We shall discuss a number of them.

Studies of physician's problem-solving

The most important and ambitious 'real-life' study on medical problem-solving is, unquestionably, that by Elstein, Shulman and Sprafka (1978). In a 'high fidelity' simulation 24 physicians interrogated three 'patients', actors, each of them playing a different role. The physicians were allowed to collect data in any sequence they wished. The actor had no fixed script beyond the opening statement of the chief complaint. Data beyond the verbal mode, e.g., physical examination, laboratory results, etc., were provided by an assistant. Between medical history and the provision of the other data a 'natural break' was provided. The scene was videotaped for reasons of 'stimulated recall', a method in which the candidate is confronted with a playback of his procedure (s) and is stimulated (by an interviewer) to think aloud about each step of the replayed videotape.

The structure of the task, the elements and characteristics of the three diseases were only briefly communicated in the book. The determination about the relevance of a certain symptom to a disease or a hypothesis (so-called 'cue') was delegated to a judging committee of experts. Unfortunately, neither explicit criteria for the relevance (weights of a cue) of the symptoms nor the number of items in the task structure were described.

Elstein *et al.* used three units of analysis of the process: information search units, cues and hypotheses. The information search units were all elements that sought information or instructed patients regarding their present or previous illness(es) of psychical or social background. Symptoms asked by a physician which were – apparently – not related to any diagnosis or hypothesis within the scope of the experimenters were listed in a different manner. Hypotheses, although not defined, served as stepping stones which could be manipulated by specific questions towards a satisfactory diagnosis.

The process was supposed to proceed along a logical, sequential line. This is in conformity with the description of hypotheses being manipulated by specific questions ('cues') but contrary to the observation that hypotheses, generated during the work-up gave the impression of hunches induced by relatively few data; they did not follow a progressively narrowing line as might have been expected in a deductive reasoning process. Nevertheless, Elstein and colleagues proposed this 'hypothetico-deductive' method as 'a nearly universal characteristic of human thinking in complex, poorly defined environments'.

As was discussed in Chapter II this 'hypothetico-deductive' method must actually be conceived of as an inductive type of reasoning. Appreciated as such it can more easily explain the outcomes of the study. The paucity of the results can partly be explained by the absence of a clear definition of the hypothetico-deductive method. Subsequently, the determination of the landmarks, which are necessary tools for the observation of the processes, suffers in consistency. Methods can greatly influence outcomes.

One of the major achievements of the Elstein *et.al.* study is the approach adopted, the development and the methodology of a simulation study of medical problem- solving. Their 'high-fidelity' simulation model proved to be a sound basis for this type of investigation.

Another major achievement was the insight generated in the course of hypotheses during the work-up. First of all there is the hypothesis generation early in the work-up of the case. These hypotheses have, as was expected, not a broad and vague character but are closely circumscribed, which must be attributed to an associative process with materials of past knowledge stored in memory. The other hypotheses generated during the work-up of the case did not follow the logical, sequential system of the first one. The investigators found the performances of the physicians to be case specific, which is a substantiation of the Newell and Simon theory about the adaptation of the individual to the problem.

The propositions of Newell and Simon were, however, explicitly made for rational human problem-solving, in the framework of 'objective' or 'accessible' knowledge as contrasted to 'personal' or 'tacit' knowledge. In the former type of reasoning one can expect a deductive outcome of the inference process, in the latter type an inductive one.

Whether the case-dependency is also valid for problem-solving processes within the sphere of 'personal' knowledge application is an open question. As our investigation is directed towards both these ways of reasoning, the matter of case-dependency shall be given attention in our chapter on results.

We reported that there is virtually no provision of schemata, particularly general schema in medicine. It often places experimenters in a difficult position, because frameworks for the observation of medical processes are not provided for by medicine itself. It leaves the investigator to produce his own models and schema for observing strategies in the clinical problem-solving processes. Apart from the reported Elstein *et al.* problem-solving strategy to our knowledge only Kleinmuntz and Kleinmuntz (1981) specified another two types of problem-solving strategy.

(a) Heuristic decision strategy: it uses heuristics to arrive at a diagnosis and then picks an acceptable treatment. This strategy considers people as satisfiers, who indulge in limited amounts of search, until a satisfactory rather than an optimal solution is reached (see Simon's Satisficing theory). The general procedure is to develop a hypothesis about the patient's disease and to try to confirm the hypothesis. It assumes that only positive evidence is sought.

(b) Generate and test strategy: it is a concise itinerary of the former strategy. The problem solver does not even bother about symptoms and signs but chooses a treatment that happens to come by.

And we can surely fall in behind Lusted (1976), who wished: 'One could hope that a small group of problem solving strategies would underly all medical diagnosis and treatment. However, if such strategies exist they are not yet understood.'

The validity of clinical judgements

Hippocrates advises us: 'From all the symptoms taken together one should form a judgement'. The comprehensive acquisition of the observable phenomena induces a judgement' a judgement which can be conceived as an object of thought. The validity of the judgement is primarily based on the physician's observation and evaluation of the diseased state of the patient.

When we want to try to get some insight into the physician's problem-solving, clinical judgement can be rated as the foremost attribute desired in physicians. The task of a physician is to render a judgement, usually a diagnostic classification or therapeutic plan, on the basis of a set of data provided by the patient. Clinical judgements are a major determinant of quality in medical practice. They enable us to evaluate the accuracy and the intellectual process of the physician's activities.

Clinical judgement is an important human cognitive activity, typically carried out by a professional person, with the aim of the prediction of significant outcomes in the life of another individual. It is suggested that the clinical judgement of a physician is, at the very least, related to his underlying intellectual ability, to the quality of his medical education and to the depth of his clinical experience. Clinical experience in particular has been viewed by physicians as being the better part of medical knowledge in making adequate judgements.

It has been claimed that knowledge gained on the basis of years of clinical experience is not reducible to explicit rules, recipes, or basic principles (Engelhardt *et al.*, 1979). However, such judgements are significantly influenced by knowledge of the outcomes. Even some data and the notion of frequency evokes the physician's judgement on only a few alternative outcomes. This is, according to Mason and Bulgren (1964), the experience of which physicians are proud. This is what appears to be the artistic ability in the practice of medicine and why it may seem to many physicians that they are gifted in making correct decisions without definable data and why they profess that rare diagnoses can be correctly made when no statistician would dare stick his neck out on the basis of the data.

According to Komaroff (1979), the rather low validity of clinical judgements may be attributed to the disturbingly 'soft' medical data. These data are defined, collected, and interpreted with a degree of variability and inaccuracy which falls short of the standard which (knowledge) engineers expect from most data. Variability in the medical history may stem from the patient's description of his illness, the physician's conduct of the interview, or the dynamic interaction between the patient and the physician during the course of the interview. The physician's conduct may be reflected in his selection of questions to ask.

Physicians, however, believe that they can 'sense' the accurate cues in a noisy environment of 'soft' data. They suggest that they are accustomed to these 'soft' data and are able to apply their clinical strategy to the case at hand. However, cognitive research pleads against them. Physicians tend to mould their configurations of symptoms and diseases to their own knowledge and opinions. They translate their knowledge into personal degrees of association between symptoms and diagnoses. These notions are reflected in clinical practice, where different (groups of) doctors will assign different diagnostic labels to the same patient.

Nobrega et al. (1977) found that doctors differed very much in recording patients' items, which can be attributed to differential knowledge, but also to differing definitions of the same situation. With Dowling (1982) we believe the latter explanation to be the more plausible one.

However, it is not the data, which constitute the judgement, but the preliminary judgement (hypothesis) which determines the acquisition and quality of the data. Barrows and Bennet (1972) were amazed that among almost all physicians the judgement was reached before all the available data from the patient had been obtained. But the doctor is quite satisfied when the acquired data satisfactorily verifies his preliminary judgement. Besides, how can a physician in a real life situation know that he has obtained all the data? How can a physician distinguish relevant from irrelevant data? How can he memorize these data? Kleinmuntz (1968) demonstrated that data not related to the physician's mental hypothesis or diagnosis are totally forgotten by the physician. During physician-patient interviews doctors often ask the same questions twice or thrice, and cease to inquire further when a stereotype pattern has come to mind. With a marginally verified pattern the doctor is quite satisfied and certain about his judgement.

Oskamp (1965) found that judges' certainty about their decisions is entirely disproportionate to the actual correctness of those decisions. The increasing feelings of confidence as the clinician works through a case are not a sure sign of increasing accuracy of his conclusions.

Goldberg (1968) comes to the conclusion that clinical judgements are:
(a) rather unreliable;
(b) minimally related to confidence and amount of experience;
(c) relatively unaffected by the amount of information available;
(d) rather low in validity.

It is because of the rather pessimistic view on the low validity of clinical judgement, and the relation to the optimization of medical care, that some people have turned to a search for a more objective way of investigating and assessing clinical judgements.

Summary

It is argued that human beings do not always act at the highest level of thinking, the level of abstract reasoning. Indeed, we shall present the opinion that most human beings, like physicians, mostly operate on a more concrete level of thinking, in order to meet the stresses and competitions to which they are exposed in real life. This thought is strengthened by the capacities of and restrictions on the thinking processes. The capacity of information processing is limited by a kind of funnel, the so-called short term memory, which acts as a gateway to an immense 'long term memory'. These limits are defined in the, called after Miller, channel capacity, which permits the processing of only a few 'bits', or items of information. This limitation can only be conquered by combining bits into 'chunks', a personal and circumstantial arrangement of bits into a pattern. These patterns act as memory elements each with its own vector that can bring them back into awareness. Any hierarchical ordering of these patterns seem to be coincidental.

Apart from channel capacity humans voluntarily limit information by simplifying the problem to comprehensible sizes, and by 'massing of data', combining several similar circumstances into one element to be remembered, in order to economize the capacity of thought. People live in a world overloaded with information. They need some devices at least to protect themselves from these information flows.

All these processes question, as a matter of course, the validity of inference. Human judgement is often less reliable as we would wish. The limited possibilities to retrace one's inferences must be viewed as a serious drawback in all judgemental situations in which we have to rely on these limping inferences.

In problem-solving mankind faces his challenge. It is one of a human's most laborious tasks. Doctors are confronted with problems daily. Sometimes it is difficult to manage these problems as they are all phrased in very personal and circumstantial ways. From this information the physician has to conceive some opinion about the patient's condition, which he tries to solve according, apparently, to certain idiosyncratic rules. However, these rules are basically a part of his task environment which creates the problem space, i.e., the combination of knowledge and application rules, in which he has to find a resolution. The strong impression exists that physicians, like other human beings, find their way to a solution by means of (repeated) pattern recognition, by some kind of 'trial and error' method.

The studies thus far on the subject of medical problem-solving have not reached definite conclusions, although a number of ideas have been presented. As we have no knowledge of the processes which underly the physician's problem-solving activities, any decision about the quality of the physician's judgement would seem to be premature.

It is our aim to clarify some of these processes as they take place in the clinical office.

Chapter IV

Clinical decision-making

Where is the wisdom we lost in knowledge?
Where is the knowledge we lost in information?
T.S. Eliot

Introduction

Decision theory has been developed from the rational economic man concept which originated during the 18th century. Under the influence of the British philosopher and economist John Stuart Mill the Utilitarian principle was introduced. It was, however, Von Neumann and Morgenstern (1947) who laid the scientific basis for decision-making. They introduced mathematical-statistical axioms and probabilistic calculations into the model which would facilitate logical reasoning while maximizing profit and minimizing costs, based on (subjective) expected utility. Utility is the value attached to the outcome of a decision process. By ordering one's preferences for the outcomes of the various alternative tracks in the process one could, by means of probabilistic calculations, choose the track with the highest gain. A number of conditions have to be fulfilled. Such axioms and conditions together constitute the rules for optimizing decision strategies. Such a model may serve as an explanation for particular processes of human thinking in the setting of a rational task environment.

However, the model developed a life of its own and was transformed from an originally descriptive model (see above) into a prescriptive one. The successors of Von Neumann and Morgenstern were no longer interested in how people behave but in how they ought to behave. They introduced more sophisticated statistical systems into the model. The most important was Bayes' formula, now two hundred years old but still very much alive. This formula is basically meant to predict future events on the basis of a (substantial) experience of the past. However, prediction is always difficult even with Bayes' formula, but it seems to be most reliable with large numbers. Large numbers, unfortunately, are seldom available in the medical world.

A large number of medical decision-making systems based on probability calculations and a very few on symbolic logic (artificial intelligence) became available to aid physicians who preferred to behave rationally in front of the patient. The results of these systems were disappointing and many people found the critically prescriptive attitude towards doctors' decision-making inherent in their theoretical prescriptive assumptions unacceptable. These systems have not been accepted on a large scale in the medical world.

Successes have been very few and, therefore, I would suggest a re-orientation of research on clinical decision-making. Decision-making is a very important feature in the clinical practice. Any improvement in understanding of these processes would not only enhance clinical judgements but could also enhance education.

Several alternative decision-making models have been developed, high-lighting a number of characteristics which are very recognizable to every physician who struggles daily with patients' problems. Since these alternatives are mainly explanatory and do not possess as yet the simplicity and intellectual force of the Von Neumann and Morgenstern theory, they can only serve as a significant initial contribution to new explorations in the fields of (clinical) decision-making.

Historical background

Humans make decisions, a tremendous number everyday, consciously or unconsciously, ranging from small ones, 'how do I like my egg in the morning?' to large ones, 'how many million dollars to invest in an uncertain business prospect?'; from the move of a chess player to the general's decision to sacrifice the lives of several hundred soldiers. Most of these decisions are based on intuition or 'common sense', or on what is assumed to be a more reliable basis, namely experience. The various unsatisfactory outcomes, not to mention disasters, resulting from this kind of decision-making, have motivated people to look for strategies yielding more acceptable outcomes, and ways were sought to develop and define strategies which would enable us to predict more reliably the outcomes of our decisions.

Cramer and Bernoulli were the first who, in the 17th and 18th century, began with the rational economic man concepts; a rational actor who behaved logically and was guided by mathematical constructs. However, their ideas did not progress very far at that time.

People still continue to lose their money in the various gambling houses in the world, to the intense joy and pleasure of the owners of these houses. The very complicated mathematical statistical procedures demanded by the above approaches prevent their routine application in these types of decision-making situations. These various theories and procedures remained dormant until the introduction of the computer which made the calculation of the proposed formulae much easier and quicker. The Second World War accelerated the process, and in the 'fourties and 'fifties of this century, a 'revival' of 'decision theory' was apparent.

The first applications of the theory to practical situations were in the areas of warfare and economics. In the next decades the theory and its various modifications were applied and tested in other fields of science including medicine. It is against this background that medical decision-making developed as an independent discipline with little relationship to the actual process of medical practice, only using 'medicine' only as a means to test the theory.

Towards a decision theory

Decision theory is a group of related constructs that seek to describe or prescribe how individuals or groups of people choose a course of action when faced with several alternatives and a variable amount of knowledge about the determinants or the outcomes of those alternatives (Albert, 1978). The theory is originally based on Mill's utilitarian principle which can be loosely summarized as: 'People strive to maximize their pleasure and to minimize their pain'; or in economic terms: 'they strive for the highest gain with minimal costs'.

The theory states that in order to reach this goal one has to follow a number of rules. In order to find and define these rules the successive investigators turned to the original rational economic man concepts of the 18th century. As the rules in these concepts are based on statistics in gambling situations, the fundamentals of decision theory are still found to lie in probability theory. The Hungarian mathematician Von Neumann laid the foundation with his book '*Zur Theorie der Gesellschaftsspiele*'[1] in 1928. A more definite theory emerged when Von Neumann combined his talents with the Austrian economist Morgenstern and they reported the results of their joint efforts in the historic book '*Theory of games and economic behaviour*' (1947). Many of the principles of decision theory stem from these authors. We shall retrace some of their thoughts, those which have particular relevance to applications in the medical context.

The starting-point for Von Neumann and Morgenstern is that most elements and questions in a decision-making process are normally stated in a qualitative fashion. As science can never be based on qualitative notions it is 'therefore necessary to formulate them (the composing elements) in quantitative terms, so that all the elements of the qualitative descriptions are taken into consideration'. To this end utility theory is adopted as a leading principle. However, as they state cautiously, 'Utility theory is taken as opportunistic'.

Some thoughts on utility theory

As the objective of utility theory is the maximization of the utilities, these values are the key features of this theory. A utility is a value that can be assigned to an outcome of a decision process. The maximum utility depends on the number of variables and the nature of the functions to be maximized. It is stated that all variables can assume any number of values. Uncontrollable variables sometimes intervene in the process. When they are purely statistical phenomena they can be eliminated. However, the most disturbing and intervening variable is man himself.

Von Neumann and Morgenstern were aware of this conflict. They state: 'No matter intervening circumstances, whether or not approached in probabilistic terms (no modus procedendi can be correct), the question of human behavior has to be approached with the attempt to understand the principle of conflict-

[1] On theory of games.

ing interests of participants/individuals'. The understanding of the decision-maker's behaviour, the apprehension of his intellectual processes, is a prerequisite to the process of reliable decision-making. In business both players, the entrepreneur and the customer, have their own interests and own approaches to a decision. The fact that every participant is influenced by the anticipated reactions of the other to his own measures, and that this is true for each of the participants, is most strikingly the crux of the matter. The personal interests and considerations of the participants cannot be caught in probabilistic terms or calculations unless we are able to discover the basic features of the intellectual processes, and to rationalize them. Every participant (in the game of economic trade) can determine the variables which describe his own actions but not those of others. Nevertheless, those 'alien' variables cannot be described by statistical assumptions because interest can run parallel as well as in opposition. The authors realize that serious barriers are set to the application of statistical methods for the quantification of the variables, because objective probability theory requires among others large numbers of observations.

This perspective is reflected by the authors as follows: 'The problem must be formulated, solved and understood for small numbers of participants before anything can be proved about the change of its character in any limiting case of large numbers'.

Von Neumann and Morgenstern formulate their overall goals as follows: 'We wish to find the mathematically complete principles which define 'rational behavior' for the participants in a social economy, and to derive from them the general characteristics of that behavior. And while the principles ought to be perfectly general – i.e. valid in all situations – we may be satisfied if we can find solutions, for the moment, in some characteristic special cases'. The restriction to these cases is: 'Since we want to theorize about 'rational behavior' there seems to be no need to give the individual advice as to his behavior in situations other than those which arise in a rational community'. The authors made clear that what might be recommendable to a (large) group does not necessarily apply to the individual. In medicine, with its individualised approaches to decision-making, serious consideration is to be given to this restraint.

We have described these assumptions in some detail because we have the impression that many successors of Von Neumann and Morgenstern do not always respect the reservations made by the founders of decision theory. The reader can deduce from these quotations that the application of decision theory in medicine will meet several obstacles. Some of these problems, like the quantification of utilities and the demands for large numbers, are still unresolved.

Before we outline some of the basic principles of utility theory some comments are called for. It becomes clear from the above analysis that utility theory, as a main foundation for decision theory, is just another model for explaining thinking processes with the restriction that it will only apply to rational processes in a utilitarian environment. Although decision theory has severely restricted its domain of study, nevertheless it can provide a valuable contribution to the study of thinking and problem-solving processes in human beings. The expansion of decision theory beyond its original borders can only be justified when the theory (and its adherents) adapts itself to the neighbouring theories of problem-solving and the behaviour of people acting in different task environments. Any claim of decision theory to provide *the* model for decision-making in general is unjustified and never was justified.

People have to make decisions, i.e., to choose between a number of alternatives. The choice can be between two or more eligible objects or between a desirable object and its costs. But comparing, which is inherent in choice, includes a system of preferences which is all-embracing and complete, i.e., for any two objects or rather for any two imagined events, the individual possesses a clear intuition of preference. It is evident that people express their preferences in a somewhat implicit way, as some kind of feeling or sensation. Utility theory tries to make explicit what in its nature is implicit. The basis of utility theory is the immediate sensation of preferences of one object or group of objects as against another. The assignment of numerical values to these preferences (utilities) provides a basis for explicitness. We become aware of the preference ordering when there is a possibility to compare the differences in utilities.

These objects or events must as a matter of course be mutually exclusive, so that no possibility of being complementary or the like exists. We shall elucidate this principle with an example given by Von Neumann and Morgenstern.

'If an individual prefers the consumption of a glass of tea (B) to that of a cup of coffee (A), and the cup of coffee to a glass of milk (C). If we now want to know whether the last preference – i.e., difference in utilities – exceeds the former, it suffices to place him in a situation when he must decide this: Does he prefer a cup of coffee to a glass the content of which will be determined by a 50–50% chance device as tea or milk. If this standpoint is accepted, then there is a criterion with which to compare the preference of C over A with preference A over B. It is well known that thereby utilities – or rather differences of utilities – become numerically measurable'.

The authors relate this type of measurement to the Euclidian calculation of points on a line. Preferences are numerical measurements for the 'distances' between the utility differences. From this it may be clear that the relationship between the various outcomes (preferences) must be linear and the completeness can be examplified by the uninterruption of the line. 'If such a numerical valuation of utilities exists at all, then it is determined up to a linear transformation' (Von Neumann and Morgenstern). The essence of utility is the relation 'greater', which can be a basis for assigning probabilities.

Von Neumann and Morgenstern lay down four (other) prerequisites:

(1) 'We have assumed only one thing, namely that imagined events can be combined with probabilities';
(2) 'Probability is interpreted as frequency in long runs'.
(3) 'The procedure for a numerical measurement of the utilities of the individual depends, of course, upon the hypothesis of completeness in the system of individual preferences'.
(4) 'If the individual's preferences are all comparable, then we can obtain a

(uniquely defined) numerical utility'. Von Neumann and Morgenstern extend this latter postulate as follows: 'We have not obtained any basis for a comparison, quantitatively or qualitatively, of the utilities of different individuals'.

From these assumptions two axioms have been defined which run as follows.

Given a relationship between two or more preferences for events (i.e., outcomes) then

- a complete ordering of the events can be given;   (Axiom 1)
- the combining of events does not interfere with ordering.   (Axiom 2)

Corrolaries to these steps are:

- it is irrelevant in which order the constituents are named, because they are alternative events;
- it is irrelevant whether a combination of two constituents is obtained in two successive steps;
- individuals can order the outcomes of their decision-making process in terms of preferences;
- complete information has been obtained;
- the ordering is based on complete information: ('The complete answer to any specific problem consists not in finding a solution, but in determining a set of all solutions', Von Neumann and Morgenstern);
- ordering allows for the assignment of numerical values in terms of probabilities;
- linear transformation allows for transitiveness of preferences (when A is preferred to B and B to C then A is also preferred to C). The linear transformation excludes the introduction of intervening variables. The choice between two types of surgery for a particular patient may not be influenced by the recent introduction of a pertinent drug;
- the outcomes or events shall be mutually exclusive;
- where case constituents are obtained in different steps they shall be independent;
- there must be something to decide upon.

It means that in a decision-making situation, e.g., deciding on treatment, a group of individuals express their preferences to the outcomes of actions in a random ordering. All possible outcomes are incorporated into this set of preferences. The outcomes must be mutually exclusive, i.e., two different drugs which only differ in their dosage cannot be included in the system. In order to be comparable the values of the preferences must be uniform. This uniformity can take any form, for instance money, but utility theory demands probability as the standard. Because of the corrolaries of probability theory the components of the set must be independent and complete. When all conditions have been fulfilled the ordering can be performed and numerical values can be assigned to each outcome. As numerical values allow for ranking the action with the highest ranking (maximum utility) can be chosen as the most optimal action. Having established this utility ranking decision theory can delineate the optimal way to reach that maximal profit.

All this will lead, according to Von Neumann and Morgenstern, to 'Standards of behavior which can be translated as a set of rules for each participant, telling him how to behave in every possible situation of the game'.

This is exactly the object that decision theory aims at. It has to provide rules, strategies, to human decision makers of whatever discipline, which will enhance the outcomes of their decision-making process, the maximization of the utilities.

Decision theory

Decision theory is a complex, somewhat ill-defined body of knowledge developed by mathematicians, economists, and psychologists attempting to prescribe how decisions should be made and to describe systematically what variables affect decision (Rapoport and Wallsten, 1972).

Decision-making can be defined as the process of thought and action involving an irrevocable allocation of resources that culminates in choice behaviour. In making a decision, a decision maker is dealing with environments, characterized by risks, uncertainty, complexity, changes over time and conflict (Sage, 1981).

The decision maker invariably has to choose from among a number of alternatives, either diagnoses or therapeutic actions. The quality of a decision depends upon how well the decision-maker is able to acquire information, to analyse the information, and to evaluate and interpret information so as to discriminate between relevant and irrelevant bits of data; it also depends upon how well the decision maker is able to cope with the stress which is invariably encountered in important decision-making circumstances (Sage, 1981). It is essentially for human decision makers to bring order into their information acquiring and processing activities, when confronted with an excess of information, unreliable information or a lack of sufficient information.

As utility theory is the leading principle of decision theory many of its conceptual components can be retraced in decision theory, like;

(a) 'the set of states of nature' (or outcomes of actions) is assumed to form a mutually exclusive and exhaustive listing of those aspects of nature which are relevant to this particular choice problem and about which the decision maker is uncertain. Uncertainty is an innate characteristic of all decision-making situations as a result of there being a problem of choice. When one can acquire a certain object without any cost, it surely does not create an uncertainty situation. When for a particular disease only one treatment is available there cannot be a choice problem.

(b) The theory postulates that when two different states, i.e., healthy or ill state of a patient, are related to the same outcome for a given action they will be labeled the same. In order to fulfil the transitiveness postulate the states must be defined in a standard terminology in order to fit a preferential ordering.

(c) The set of possible actions and outcomes is finite, complete, and invariant for a given problem. Incompleteness makes preferential ordering illusory. The factors that are absent can be the most preferred outcome; or a new action can lead to different outcomes, etc. When a doctor is choosing between a surgical and a radiological treatment and suddenly a new drug treatment becomes available during the decision process, this latter treatment cannot become part of this decision process.

Invariableness for a given problem is another prerequisite to rational decision-making. When a particular action leads to varying results estimations and calculations become impossible. In a similar way the 'given problem' must be invariable too. When a diagnosis does not invariably mean the same thing, the application of decision theory becomes fallacious.

(d) The optimal solution depends directly on the probability assignments (weightings to the component elements of the state of nature). In the medical world the probabilistic values must come from (large) groups of patients with the same disease in a circumscribed population. In order to fulfil the conditions of objective probability theory these groups must contain a sufficient number of elements (patients), consistent in several aspects, and the elements must be randomly distributed in the population. Only in a (very) small number are these probabilistic values available.

(e) The sum of the probability of all outcomes for a given action must be unity. This also is a prerequisite of probability calculus.

(f) Sometimes a sixth component is added.
The probability assignment reflect the confidence of the decision maker in the likelihood of outcomes. In our opinion this additional statement contradicts the postulates of Von Neumann and Morgenstern as it introduces subjective probability into the system. It is exactly here that differences of conception with regard to decision theory appear.

These features specify completely the decision-making model assuming that the decision maker acts rationally.

The decision maker becomes aware of a problem, studies it, carefully weighs alternative means to a solution and makes a choice or decision guided by an objective set of values. It implies that:

(a) the decision maker is confronted with an issue that can be meaningfully isolated from other issues;

(b) objectives are identified, structured, and weighed according to their importance in satisfying specific needs;

(c) possible activities to resolve needs are identified;

(d) the utility of each alternative is evaluated in terms of its impact upon needs; and

(e) the utilities of all alternatives are compared and the policy with the highest utility is selected for action implementation.

Generally, two types of rational decision-making models are distinguished.

(A) Sequential.

(B) Dynamic.

In the former type the stage-to-stage change in the state of the system does *not* depend on the decision maker's previous decisions.

In the dynamic type the stage-to-stage changes are directly affected by the decision maker's previous decisions. In the dynamic decision model the sequence of decisions is taken in advance; the sequential theory is more concerned with the logically prior problem of diagnosis. Especially in the medical diagnostic sphere is the sequential type by far the more prevalent one.

As the rules of the decision-making process in the rational actor model are based on mathematical-statistical conceptions, medical diagnosis also has to be understood in these terms. Rapoport and Wallsten (1972) define diagnosis 'as the process of revising a subjective probability over a set of (. .) events on the basis of some data. Formally, these events are probabilistic distributions. Bayes' rule provides the mathematically appropriate way to combine the events (probability distributions) with the prior probabilities after a number of observations to obtain the posterior probabilities'.

Translated to the medical world it says: suppose we have on the basis of some data a certain idea about a particular hypothesis of a particular disease of which we know its particular prevalence (frequency in a population). Each acquired symptom or sign relevant to the disease represents an event, a step. The degree of relevancy of a symptom to the disease can be defined as a probability, a chance. With each step the original prior probability will be changed, until we finally arrive at a diagnosis, which is, as a matter of course, also assigned by a probability. After we have acquired the relevant data, this probability is called the posterior probability. The total sum of posterior probabilities for the same disease is the basis for the prior probability of the next patient (the new prior probability is computed from the old prior $+ 1$, i.e., the new diagnosis).

This probabilistic exercise is executed by means of the so-called Theorema of Bayes. Because of its important role in the process, this process is often referred to as 'Bayesian revision of opinion'.

Before considering the critically important limitations assumed by the Bayesian approach let us first consider the rule itself.

Bayes' Theorem

The reverend Thomas Bayes, an English minister, who lived from 1702 to 1761, wrote 'An essay towards solving a problem in the doctrine of chances', which was communicated to the Royal Academy of Science by his friend, Mr. Price. In an introduction to the essay Bayes wrote 'that his design at first in thinking on the subject of it was, to find out a method by which we might judge concerning the probability that an event has to happen, in given circumstances, upon supposition that we know nothing concerning it but that, under the same circumstances, it has happened a certain number of times, and failed a certain other number of times'. 'This problem is by no means merely a curious speculation in the doctrine of chances, but necessary to be solved in order to (provide) a sure foundation for all our reasonings concerning past facts, and what is likely to be hereafter'.

Given the number of times in which an unknown event has happened and
failed, the problem can be defined as:
>   the chance that the probability of its happening in a single trial lies
>   somewhere between any two degrees of probability that can be named.

Bayes stated the following definitions:
(1)   Several events are inconsistent, when, if one of them happens, none of
      the rest can.
(2)   Two events are contrary when one, or other of them must, and both
      together, cannot happen.
(3)   An event is said to fail when it cannot happen, or (which comes to the
      same thing), when its contrary has happened.
(4)   An event is said to be determined when it either happened or failed.
(5)   The probability of any event is the ratio between the value at which an
      expectation depending on the happening of the event ought to be
      computed, and the value of the thing expected upon its happening.
(6)   By chance is meant the same as probability.
(7)   Events are independent when the happening of any one of them does
      neither increase nor abate the probability of the rest.
In the first four definitions Bayes defined the events and their relationships.
In definition seven the requirement of independence is added to definition
five.

Essential to Bayes' Theorem is the notion of the conditional probability: the
probability of an event given another event, not contradicting the former one.
It involves two events, with the occurrence of the second event depending on
the previous occurrence of the first. This is summarized as the probability of a
symptom or sign or test given a disease-entity, ($P[S:D]$). This means that in an
arrangement of two sets of elements, S and D, in a finite population, we are
interested in the intersection of the sets S and D, diagrammatically shown in a
Venn diagram (see, e.g., Feinstein, 1977; Wulff, 1976).

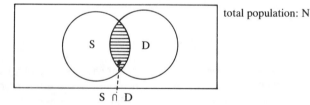

total population: N

$S \cap D$

When we read for S symptom or sign and D disease, then the intersection
$S \cap D$ means that the (set of) symptom(s) is fully compatible with disease D (or
set of diseases). After Yerushalmy and Palmer (1959) we call this probability
segment of true symptoms given the disease: Sensitivity, which is denoted as
$p[S/D]$. The other sections can also be denoted in terms of conditional probability as can easily be read from the diagram. (A non-symptom existence and
a non-diseased state is denoted in lower case letters.)

$p[D]$ is the probability of a diseased population in a total population N: the prevalence;

$p[S]$ is the probability of a (set of) symptoms prevalent in the total population N;

$P[s/D]$ false negative rate;

$P[s/d]$ specificity;

$P[S/d]$ false positive rate.

As the section can never be more or less than its total size, the probability of a particular section always amounts to 1.0 (e.g., all the probabilities of the various figures on a dice together come to 1.0). So the section S is represented by

$$p[S/D] + p[S/d] = 1 \text{ or: } p[S/D] + 1\text{-}p[S/D],$$

and for the negative side

$$p[s/d] + p[s/D] = 1 \text{ or: } p[s/d] + 1\text{-}p[s/d].$$

The elements of the formula thus having been sketched we now come to the theorema itself. The formula can be approached in the classical form of subjective or inductive probability (see chapter II, probabilistic reasoning). We there formulated our question as: 'What are your estimates of getting a six in the next cast with a dice?'. The answer was 0.5 as we were only interested in obtaining a six or a non-six (compare 'having a disease or non-disease').

$$p[6] = \frac{6}{6 + (\text{non-6})} .$$

Bayes' formula can be denoted as the sum of the probability of all favourable events relevant to a state divided by the probability of all events favourable and the probability of non-favourable events relevant to a state. In conformity with the denotation in the Venn diagram Bayes' formula can be depicted as

$$p[D/S] = \frac{p[S/D \times p[D]}{p[S/D] \times p[D] + p[S/d] \times p[d]}$$

$p[D/S]$ being the predictive value for having the disease given the (set of) symptoms. or in words

$$\text{Predictive value} = \frac{\text{Sensitivity} \times \text{Prevalence}}{\text{Sensitiv.} \times \text{Preval.} + (1\text{-Specificity}) \times (1\text{-Preval.})} .$$

The particular feature of Bayes' theorem is that it strives to combine the two types of statistical probabilities: the objective and subjective probabilities. The basic principle of Bayes' theorem is that it tries to provide prediction from the relative frequencies of success. The larger the success rate the greater the chance that the prediction 'p' approaches the success rate 'r', so that in the end the equation is 'p' = 'r'. This means that the inferred (subjective) probabilities have values close to the relative (objective) frequency value (n_1/n, 'n_1' being the successes and 'n' the total population). But that is exactly what we infer in inductive reasoning: the more we have seen a white swan the more we believe all swans to be white; the more we have seen patients with influenza, the more we believe the next patient will have influenza. Bayes' formula represents the classical problem of induction: to estimate the probability that an event will occur in the future on the basis of its frequency of occurrence in the past (Simon, 1957).

It does not mean that Bayes' formula is invalid. The formula can provide a substantial contribution to the probabilistic approach of rational decision-making, when account is taken of the correct conditions. It is not, however, in conformity with the assumptions of the logically deductive rational actor model of Von Neumann and Morgenstern.

For the appropriate application of Bayes' theorem not in general but to medicine in particular, a number of requirements must be fulfilled.

The most important are:

(a) a set of reasonable beliefs can be represented by a probability function defined over propositions 'S' and 'D'; reasonable changes of belief can be represented by a process called 'conditionalization', i.e., construction of new statement in terms of conditional probabilities (Tautu and Wagner, 1978). It is believed that these beliefs and their changes can be expressed in numerical terms.

(b) The measures reflect the opinions of ideally consistent people.

(c) The particular set of diseases should be well-defined, so that the frequency of characters in the individual diseases and the frequency of these diseases in the particular population under study are known (Baron and Fraser, 1965). It requires that this population, or sample size, is actually known, and of sufficient size to permit satisfactory estimation. The actual performance of a Bayesian calculation is difficult, because it depends on quantitative data that are seldom available. To apply Bayes' theorem one has to make use of personal judgements of more or less experienced physicians about these probabilities. The drawbacks to this procedure have been sketched elsewhere (see Chapter I).

(d) The diagnoses used must constitute a complete diagnostic system, i.e., be mutually exclusive and together cover all possible diagnoses (Salamon et al., 1976). Mutual exclusivity is only rarely to be found when the physician is presented with the patient's chief complaint (Pauker and Szolovits, 1977).

(e) To make any scientific sense the Bayesian approach should encounter and set the task context for the essential determinants of the judgemental process. Research suggests that it does not (Kahnemann and Tversky, 1972).

(f) Posterior binomial estimates have to be determined by sample difference rather than sample proportion. In subjective probability estimation people tend to react in a reverse way. They also do not depend on the population proportion. In his evaluation of evidence, man is apparently not a conservative Bayesian (as is often believed): he is not Bayesian at all (Kahnemann and Tversky, 1972).

(g) Bayesian inference is aimed at specific diagnoses and actions, not at the uncertain decisions of clinicians (Feinstein, 1977). In other words, it lacks reality.

(h) Each new piece of evidence acquired by research will change nomenclature, frequency distributions of disease and symptoms and their co-occurrence. It will hamper the consistent application of Bayes' theorem.

(j) The theory requires that symptoms and diseases be independent. One of the most serious statistical problems outstanding in diagnosis is that of symptom interactions (Anderson and Boyle, 1968). Norusis and Jacquez (1975a, b) presented a simple example of the importance of the joint distribution of two variables.

SCHEMA

Joint distribution of two symptoms S1, S2

	Disease 1 S1			Disease 2 S1	
	Present	Absent		Present	Absent
Present S2	0.5	0	Present S2	0	0.5
Absent	0	0.5	Absent	0.5	0

Where in both diseased states two symptoms have equal probabilities any discrimination of the diseased states would fail, although considering those states jointly would reveal that the first symptom is present in one disease with a probability of 0.5 and absent in the other, while the second symptom shows the reverse.

As we discussed in Chapter II, the notion of independence is not only a prerequisite to the application of Bayes' theorem (as Bayes himself emphasized!) but is critical to the validity of the probability calculations. Ignoring this prerequisite can lead to variable and unpredictable outcomes. Since several decision-making systems have been tested on their original own data base, which was first used in the initial matrix, this critical condition is frequently overlooked. It is precisely here that the application of the Bayesian formula to clinical decision processes falls down. The lack of a standard terminology makes any statement about the independence of medical data unverifiable and hence the entirety of calculations and conclusions questionable.

A number of variations on the Bayesian model have been proposed. Croft (1972) tested 10 of the most commonly used mathematical diagnostic models on the same large set of data. He found that their diagnostic accuracy is more sensitive to variations between the diseases than variations between the mathematical models. He recommended future researchers not to continue with increasingly sophisticated mathematical techniques, but, instead, to tackle the real obstacles to practical computer-aided medical diagnosis. These obstacles are:

(1) lack of standard medical definitions;

(2) lack of large, reliable medical data bases, and
(3) lack of acceptance of computer-aided diagnosis by the medical profession.

Croft and Machol (1974) considered medical diagnosis as a pattern-recognition problem. Confirming the suggestions of Baron and Fraser (1965), they recommended that the entire taxonomy of diseases first be studied and re-examined.

Constraints on the rational decision maker

From the preceding description of the so-called rational decision-making process a number of requirements are necessary pre-conditions to its use, namely:
(1) comprehensive identification of all relevant variables, constraints, and modifiers;
(2) determination and clarification of all relevant objectives;
(3) determination and minimization of costs and maximization of effectiveness;
(4) impartiality in probability estimation and calculation;
(5) acceptance of the assumption of transitiveness of preferences;
(6) compliance with the conditions for the application of Bayes' formula.

Given the stringent requirements it is hardly surprising that the applications are limited to a narrowly circumscribed area of clinical medicine. In the applications to clinical practice it is the treatment part of the medical process that is usually chosen. This has the advantage of starting from a clearly defined starting-point (whether true or not is not relevant), a specified diagnosis, and a limited (compared to the diagnostic part) number of relevant alternatives. The doctor defines his decision criteria, e.g., drug treatment versus surgery; he is familiar with all relevant alternatives, e.g., doing nothing (watchful expectation) or X-ray treatment; he is reasonably aware of their possible consequences and assigns to each of them a preference value representing a subjective probability to an expected outcome; he ranks the alternatives in a preferred order of rational impact; by calculating the probabilities he is able to select the alternatives which rate highest in terms of expected outcome; provided:
(i)   that the doctor has sufficient time;
(ii)   that the doctor has all the information (which he can only know with hindsight);
(iii) that the doctor has sufficient cognitive capacity.

To assist the decision maker in this comprehensive task he is encouraged to design a hierarchically structured branching tree in which the branches represent all the alternatives and the ends of the branches are the buds that can flower at various stages. A 'cue' (compare Miller's 'bits', Chapter III) is assumed to have an impact on 2 or 3 subsequent branches. Once one has focused a particular route the acquisition of cues gives the impression of the unfolding of the branches of the tree. Attaching probabilities to the cues makes it possible to combine them with the probabilistic values of the outcomes. Calculation along all the branches provides one with a set of numerical values. The subjectively estimated probabilities lead one to the highest (maximum) expected utility. This gave the theory its name: subjective expected utility theory, in short SEU.

It is easily understood that the number of cues has to be limited in order to maintain supervision over the widely (or even wildly) unfolding branching tree. Pauker and Kassirer (1980) suggest cutting a number of branches when the tree threatens to outgrow one's supervision. They suggest limiting the breadth and the length of the decision tree to the depth of 5 or 6 steps and 3 or 4 different branches. They called this procedure the 'threshold approach'. But this tactic would seriously violate the prerequisites stated in the theory. In other words, this type of decision-making, if it is possible, can only be restricted to (very) simple situations; situations in which most physicians experience no difficulty in arriving at an excellent decision, even without calculations.

The other problem we have to face in using the rational decision maker's approach is the assignment of probabilities to cues or steps in the branching tree. The availability of probability estimates in medicine is very, very limited. Only in a handful of circumstances are objective probabilities (requiring large numbers of observations!) for cue-disease relationships or prevalence rates for diseases available. Gustafson *et al.* (1971) advocated using subjective estimation of the various values by the expert physician. They defined subjective probability as any estimate of the probability of an event, which is given by a subject or inferred from his behaviour. Subjective estimates can be derived from experts, frequency data from literature or medical records or from interviewing a random sample of physicians.

But in all these recommended sources of probability estimations we have to assume an actual or conceivable sequence of events (see Chapter II) of which we cannot have any knowledge. As the experts' own backgrounds represent for the most part only a very restricted section of the total (diseased) population, their estimates may be far from true objective values. Medical literature is customarily written by experts and suffers, therefore, from the same restrictions. Grouping randomly sampled physicians (how?) cannot lead to any greater clarification because all of them have a specific sequence of events in mind: the grouping subsequently decreases the validity of their personal opinions.

However, as Kassirer (1976) points out, when literature provides unsatisfactory answers, the situation requires the 'judgment of an experienced clinician' or the application of 'common sense'. It implies reliance on personal judgement and personal intuition, because there is no evidence that the probability estimations of experts are more reliable than those of laymen. But this is putting the cart before the horse: if you want to improve the decision, do not use inadequate data. We have to acknowledge that when we screen the medical literature we come across large gaps in existing knowledge, usually suggesting the need for future research.

Furthermore, for the more accessible prior probability estimates unreliability of the estimations is the rule rather than the exception. Problems inherent

in prior probability estimations are, e.g:
  (1) the estimates discriminate against rare diseases;
  (2) prior probabilities as figures for prevalence are almost unavailable, and
       when they are, they are seldom reliable. Incidence figures are not
       available at all;
  (3) sampling errors;
  (4) estimates may only be applicable to a given population in a particular
       geographical location;
  (5) estimates can easily be distorted by seasonal and investigational influ-
       ences;
  (6) estimates may have a personal and situational emphasis. Physicians do
       not rely heavily on generally accessible knowledge like textbooks,
       journals, continuing education, etc. Many of those making estimates
       rely on direct experience with their own patients. Kochen (1983) found
       that physicians primarily rely on:
       (a) own experience : 100%;
       (b) literature   : 65%;
       (c) medical school   : 24%.

Many of the constraints the rational decision maker faces stem from two
fields: the medical and the probabilistic. The medical field suffers from a lack
of standard terminology and clear definitions (see Chapter I) while the conditions as set by probability theory are a subsequent obstacle on top of the first.
Unfortunately, these are not the last difficulties in the path of the rational
decision maker.

The most difficult and yet unresolved problem is utility estimation. Lindley
(1975) believes that 'it (the theory) is one of the great triumphs of modern
thinking to show that only by assigning such a single numerical measure
sensible decisions can be made. Only by measuring the quality of life can
rational decisions be made'. Still, it is an open question how to quantify the
quality of life and who is to quantify it. People often exhibit patterns of
preference which appear incompatible with the expected utility theory. Because of the impossibility of establishing objective criteria for measuring
someone's quality of life, one has to rely on subjective estimation.

However, Kahnemann and Tversky (1979) showed that this assumption is
violated in several ways. Generally, people overweight outcomes that are
considered certain. On the other hand, when uncertainty dominates in a
particular proposition, risk-seeking behaviour can be observed. In a choice
situation people prefer certainty to probability although the numerical outcomes may have the same (or even higher for the chance proposition) value.
For instance, when subjects were asked for their preference in a simplified case
of 50% chance to win $ 1000 or $ 450 for certain, most people prefer the latter
option (risk averse). But, when this proposition is reflected into negative
prospects (losses instead of gains) the reaction of the subjects is reversed. Risk
seeking is more prevalent in choices with assumed negative outcomes.

People normally perceive outcomes as gains or losses rather than as final
states of wealth or welfare as utility theory postulates. The appreciation of

'gain' or 'loss' is relevant to the current analysis of personal comfort (wealth or welfare). Every individual has his own 'level of appreciation' (or 'reference point') which can fluctuate for various situations. Particular influence on this 'reference point' can be demonstrated for the context in which the choice problem appears or is offered. In health care the prospects of health, disability, or death can profoundly affect people's appreciation of 'gains' or 'losses' with subsequent effect on personal 'reference points'.

This approach to choice problems may produce inconsistent preferences. Many carriers of value or utility are changes of circumstances rather than final propositions. In their prospect theory Kahnemann and Tversky (1979) made perfectly clear that people's behaviour and appreciation of probability violates the assumptions of utility theory.

As long as (i) the diagnosis is clearcut, (ii) the number of possible (therapeutic) actions – very – limited and (iii) the outcomes (as states of health) can be defined in two states: dead or alive, then the problem of utility can easily be solved. But when do we, physicians, meet such a situation? And if we meet it, do we need these uncertain calculations to govern our steps? Doctors' problems are always concerned with non-simple questions, with several possible actions, and a variety of different outcomes, largely beyond determination. Considering medical options only in terms of life and death is inadequate. People are more than a mere biological phenomenon.

Every individual estimates his own 'utility', while society may also place a numerical worth upon its members. The physician implicitly places a utility upon his patient. Whenever physicians make clinical decisions they integrate their own value system to generate preferences for alternative diagnoses, therapies and outcomes. The greater the cultural gap between patient and physician, the more difficult this appreciation of values becomes. This seems especially true for decisions under risk.

The estimation of a utility value is contingent on a specific situation, in which the preferences of the physician and the patient may be in conflict. Apart from broad categories such as life and death, and estimates of the expected survival (assuming it can be forecast), we cannot see how normative, or objective, utility estimates can be determined.

It means that for every specific process and for every specific state-of-health a generally accepted numerical value has to be established. Of course, every physician makes this type of estimation every day. Most processes share many components. Most health states have more features in common than features where they differ. Even among physicians disagreement is less than is suggested. However, people tend to disregard components that alternatives share and focus on the components that distinguish them (Tversky, 1972). They do not consider themselves as part of statistics or frequency distributions and hence emphasize their differences. Besides, computations based on subjective estimates of physicians do not make the value estimates more objective. Theories and standards applied in financial and economic disciplines cannot be transplanted to medicine as such. Analyses of preferences will often lead to ill-considered, often accidental incompleteness. Lindblom (1980, 1959) indicates

a number of limitations to such analysis:
  (a) it is fallible, never achieves infallibility, and can be poorly informed, superficial, biased, or mendacious;
  (b) it cannot wholly resolve conflicts of value and interests;
  (c) sustained analysis may be too slow and too costly compared with realistic needs;
  (d) the way an issue is formulated suggests more often the creation of a policy than a call for choice preferences.

The variability of disease characteristics, predictions, therapeutic and treatment possibilities and appreciations of health states makes the establishment of utility theory as the basis for medical decisions impractical and a normative classification of utilities illusory. According to Lindblom means and ends, treatment and outcomes, are often confounded. The identification of values and goals is not distinct from the analysis of alternative actions. Agreement on a good policy does not necessarily include that it is the most appropriate means to an end. Besides, analysis may be limited, important options neglected, and outcomes not·considered. It often seems that there is a greater preoccupation with ills to be remedied than with positive goals to be sought (Lindblom, 1959).

The changing views on health, disease and cost make normative utility valuation fallacious. What may be wisdom today, may be foolishness tomorrow.

In daily practice the estimation of the utility is most often conveniently left to the physician: 'Doctor knows what is good for me'. When the expected utility is expressed on a scale between 0 and 1, the physician invariably aims at the upper part of the scale. People expect him to react in this way. Every result below this expected outcome leads to severe disappointment and the patient urges him to search diligently for more powerful treatments. Moreover, the physician decides upon the whole of the medical process, in which each element depends on and influences the other. A physician is really amazed when he is asked to evaluate a single feature of the medical process. Besides, the personality of the physician greatly influences the estimation, as has been studied and shown by several psychologists (e.g., Tversky and Kahnemann, 1981, 1974; Lichtenstein et al., 1978; Slovic et al., 1977).

But when objective values cannot be provided and subjective utilities are unreliable, what about decision theory? De Dombal (1978) spoke about utility as 'the chief unsolved problem in medical decision making'.

Meeting the rational decision-maker

'The classical theory (of the rational economic man model) is a theory of a man choosing among fixed and known alternatives, to each of which is attached known consequences. But when perception and cognition intervene between the decision maker and his objective environment, this model no longer proves adequate. We need a description of the choice that recognizes that alternatives are not given but must be sought; and a description that takes into account the arduous task of determining what consequences will follow on each alternative' (Simon, 1959).

Obviously, from the late 'fifties onwards decision theory has drifted away from the original concept of being an explanation of decision making processes in order to provide the decision-maker with tools to maximize his output. Amazingly, the disappointing results in economics were the reason for enhancing the mathematical-statistical structure instead of studying the particular task environment and problem space of subjects. The decision-theoretical scientist seems no longer to be interested in human cognitive and psychological processes, but is completely absorbed in his own world of optimizing and maximizing utilities. But people are not interested in maximizing utility. The evidence on rational decision-making is largely negative evidence, evidence on what people do NOT do (Politser, 1981).

One of the problems of behaving rationally and in conformity with the rules of utility theory is its dependence on complex calculations. For this task the rational decision maker needs:
- sufficient time;
- sufficient information;
- sufficient cognitive capacity.

The complexity of the calculation, the time-consuming procedure and the cognitive stress were certainly serious drawbacks to any application of decision theory into real-life economic situations. The rational decision maker could not cope with such an approach when he has to act with in his own complicated task environment. Most real-life choices still lie beyond the reach of maximizing techniques – unless the situations are heroically simplified by drastic approximations (Simon, 1959). What was true for economics was certainly true for a complicated discipline such as medicine. Although the introduction of decision theory into the medical world started 10–15 years later (compared with the economic world) it met with almost the same problems as in the economic arena.

When the computer entered the scene it was warmly welcomed. Now a number of the restraints on rational decision could be tackled. The calculations, storage of data for objective probability estimations, and (parts of) information-processing were the first areas to be considered for simplification. This could all be accomplished by mankind's newest toy. It is my opinion that the introduction of the computer into the world of decision-making marked a decisive turning point. The rapidly increasing capabilities of the machine, its miniaturization, its accessibility, and availability, created tremendous possibilities for information scientists to develop highly sophisticated programmes. This led them to turn away from the potential user with his built-in restraints and fallible estimations. No longer was any adaption to the user seriously considered, but the user had to adapt to the programme (read: programme maker). Although comparisons with physicians' work are regularly made, and are spoken of as 'computer aids' for doctors, physicians are often blamed for not behaving in a 'probabilistic fashion' or 'unable to estimate probabilities and utilities', thereby suggesting that doctors should think and act in these ways. 'They violate the principles of rational decision-making when judging probabilities, making predictions, or otherwise attempting to cope with probabilistic tasks' (Slovic et al., 1977).

The scale had tilted. Information scientists assumed that their intervention was called for. 'Since doctors themselves don't take active part in it, the main thrust is carried by people coming from informatics as such. What the physician needs, if anything, is a decision support for the steps in his clinical decision, not the ultimate classification of the problems' (de Dombal and Gremy, 1976).

The Leeds computer programme for the diagnosis of acute abdomen outperforms even the senior clinicians, de Dombal *et al.* reported triumphantly in 1975. This was the big breakthrough. Medicine could now be turned into mathe-medicine. Huge clinical data bases like COSTAR, PROMIS, TMIS, CARE, ARAMIS, CASNET, etc., were installed in order to provide the computer programmers with the necessary data on prior and conditional probabilities. 'Mankind' (read: information scientists) were in need of these 'objective' probabilities and 'objective' utilities; utilities in which every health status for every individual, at every age, in every possible social status would be captured into a numerical value. Certainly, it could not take long before physicians were replaced by an interviewing, information-processing, utility and probability calculating machine. This suggestion was fervently denied by the information and computer scientists, but the fact that they first came up with this suggestion casts some doubt on their denials.

The 'seventies were characterized by the emergence of innumerable computer programs designed for decision-making in clinical practice. Piles of 'computer aids' with flowery fancy names poured out over the medical world. However, in 1977 Feinstein warned against this over-enthousiasm. 'I know', Feinstein says, 'of no published work, or clinical setting, or specific world situation, in which Bayesian methods have made a prominent contribution that could not have been achieved just as easily without the Bayes formula. Bayesian inference rests on the idea that the posterior probability of an event is proportional to the product of its prior probability multiplied by the likelihood ratio. But the Bayesian statistician does not know the prior probability. He must make a subjective, personal guess called an estimate. When Bayesian methods depend on intuitions and hunches, we only replace clinical by statistical hunches which does not bring us any step farther'. And Young (1982) stated that 'it must be clear that physicians will reject systems that dogmatically offer advice without proven benefit in allround situations even if it displays impressive diagnostic accuracy'.

Some ten years later the dream has ended. No robots in doctors' offices, no replacement of the physician, no adaption of the user to the system, but an acknowledgement by Howell (1982): 'Instead we should concentrate on what people actually do and develop descriptive models to account for decision processes'. It seems to me that after the over-enthusiastic period of the 'seventies, a period of reflection, of hesitation, has entered on the scene. Maybe researchers do not always pay enough attention to basic questions, switch the goals and the means, zealously overrun practical applications, sanctify the program more than the physician. Where computer-aided decision-making promised insight into the physician's thought processes (Pauker *et al.,* 1976) and a resulting better understanding of the human diagnostic process (Rogers *et al.,* 1979), it has thus far failed in its mission.

What went wrong? What obstacles could account for this failure? In our opinion the biggest problem for decision theory is in its tuning into the thought processes of people. Von Neumann and Morgenstern assumed that their model could simulate the thought processes of rational decision makers, but they failed to prove it. It can be assumed either that people are not rational decision makers or, on the other hand, it is possible that the model did not correctly simulate people's thinking processes. Furthermore, in the attempts to attune decision theory to clinical applications several barriers were met, among which are the following.

(1) The identification of the most relevant information. The problem is that we do not know what data is relevant prior to the analysis. A study of chest pain (Pipberger *et al.,* 1968) showed that out of 498 information items under study, 55 was the maximum required for effective differential diagnosis and nearly 90% of the total information available was either redundant ōr irrelevant both for the description of the disease entities and for the differential diagnosis. But Pipberger *et al.* could only determine these facts afterwards, not during the diagnostic process.

(2) Reproducibility of information and clear terminology. This is a fundamental issue in medical practice, as we have discussed earlier. Not only the names of diseases but also the names of symptoms can be confusing. The symptom 'dyspnea' can mean 'tightness in the chest' as well as 'afraid', 'nausea' or 'dizziness', varying with situation, time, geographical area, culture, etc. In addition, symptoms can be accompanied by a number of adjectives, e.g., whether the 'oppression' is episodic or continuous, day or night, with exertion or at rest, etc. Computer programs require the use of vocabularies that are free of ambiguity (Dudley, 1968). Unless medical science solves this problem, computer directed diagnostic aids will play only a small part in ongoing medical decision-making.

(3) Comparability of terminology. In particular, classifications and taxonomies of diseases must be revised in order to develop a uniform system for unambiguous use by all physicians throughout the world.

(4) Test optimization. The results of laboratory tests are assumed to be more solid data in clinical decision-making. However, the clinician's interpretation of the results and their connection to clinical findings is often erroneous. 'There are many reasons why clinicians misinterpret laboratory test results they need or request laboratory tests they neither need nor really use' (Zieve, 1966). Zieve listed 10 headings each containing several examples of misinterpretation of laboratory results. These headings are: (1) technical errors; (2) physiologic variation; (3) over-interpretation of test values; (4) unfamiliarity with procedures or with physiologic factors affecting them; (5) unawareness of extraneous factors that influence tests; (6) unawareness of the nature of the distri-

butions of normal; (7) uncritical acceptance of published opinions regarding the comparative value of tests supposedly measuring the same function; (8) unnecessary use of tests; (9) unnecessary repetition of tests; (10) failure to interpret tests in relation to clinical findings.

(5) Analysis of data and allocating the patients to a problem/disease class. The current taxonomic system of 'disease' is grossly unsatisfactory for both science and health care in classifying the difficulties that patients present to doctors (Feinstein, 1967). By abandoning this nomenclature and allowing each problem to be expressed in its own observational terms, Weed (1970) provided an intellectual liberation from the nosographic shackles imposed by the restricted scope of entities in the conventional taxonomy of 'disease'. But in replacing the diagnostic nomenclature of disease 'by a pragmatic nomenclature of problems, Weed has exchanged a standardized but inadequate taxonomy for an adequate but unstandardized taxonomy' (Feinstein, 1973).

(6) Limitations of problem classes. Unfortunately, the present medical taxonomy is more likely to expand its classes (e.g., with psycho-social disturbances) than to restrict them. In a study by Lipkin 21 haematological diseases were (conveniently) grouped into 9 classes, apparently chosen because the grouping reduced the time for the computer to process the data. This resulted in some remarkable appositions – e.g., of uremic anemia and acute post-haemorrhagic anemia – in the same class, while megaloblastic anemia could only be found under the headings 'pernicious anemia' and 'tropical sprue' (Scadding, 1967). This can lead to highly confusable situations.

(7) Prior and conditional probabilities. This matter has been discussed in previous sections.

(8) Stability of the probabilities. It is far from plausible that these probabilities remain stable. Changing views on health and disease, health care, medical research as well as progress in treatment possibilities make stable probabilities illusory.

(9) Quantification of utilities, and

(10) Clarification of outcome states. The problems these items pose are assumed to be insurmountable and have already been discussed.

(11) Change of symptoms during the course of the disease. In the beginning the symptom-pattern of a disease may largely differ from the pattern in a more advanced phase. This may lead to different appreciations of the diseased state of the patient by a primary care doctor and a hospital-based doctor because of time lag. In chronic diseases various phases of the disease are known to exist, each phase with its own specific pattern, and, regrettable, the phases do not always follow a strict sequential ordering.

(12) Changes in prior probabilities with seasonal or epidemic conditions.

(13) Assumption of statistical independence of each datum.

It is my opinion that we should make a fresh start in our approach to clinical decision-making. Decision-making is too important a factor in human life to waste time on impractical approaches. We have to take the decision theory perspective seriously and investigate what went wrong and look for alternative ways to assess human judgement with a view to upgrading its quality. Perhaps we must reconsider the basic principles and axioms of decision theory as it, in the modern version of the rational economic man model, was formulated by Von Neumann and Morgenstern. The principles and axioms have not fundamentally changed throughout the decades. Maybe their basic assumption of a rational decision-maker was a day-dream.

We discussed and criticised above the erroneous mixture of subjective and objective probabilities. Any assumption about the equality of both estimations leads to fallacious reasoning. In testing a theory coincidental equalities of the two types of probability cannot be conceived as a verification of the test. Furthermore, as tests are usually performed in simplified experimental environments, they cannot act as a reliable proof of a theory which pretends to simulate real life situations.

Experimenters who want to measure utilities face innumerable difficulties, which they try to avoid by confronting subjects with simple choice systems like lottery tickets or marbles in a bag at various odds. The stakes in these games are kept intentionally low. In these circumstances with a very small number of (decision) branches of a tree, the person behaves reasonably within the context of normative decision theory.

However, when these experiments are extended to more realistic situations, people divert from the predictions made by the theory. They behave in a way that is less and less consistent with the theory. This observation is also consistent with the experiments of Von Neumann and Morgenstern. Only in their least complicated experiment, the so-called zero-sum two persons game, did they find behaviour consistent with their axioms.

Rapoport and Wallsten (1972) found that risk strongly influences the actor's behaviour. Subjects are conservative in their behaviour: they estimate 'on the safe side'. Experienced people give considerably more extreme estimates than naive subjects and make their final decision on the basis of less evidence. The excellent studies of Kahnemann and Tversky (1972, 1973, 1974) and Slovic, Fischhoff, Lichtenstein (1971–1982) indicate that humans, generally speaking, are not only irrational estimators, but they are also convinced of the rationality of their estimates.

Obviously, most real life choices still lie beyond the reach of maximizing techniques – unless the situations are heroically simplified by approximations (Simon, 1959). It seems that if we want to meet the real rational decision maker we shall have to wait, and as far as my fallible estimation goes, to wait for a long, long time.

This collision between theory and reality gave rise to alternative conceptions of decision-making, which started during the late 'fifties. We shall report on them in the last section of this Chapter.

Artificial intelligence

Before reporting on the alternative decision-making models we shall first focus briefly on a development in problem-solving and decision-making which started in approximately the same era as the modern version of decision theory, namely the rise of artificial intelligence. Although the start of this discipline must be dated back to the beginning of this century, its development and application has only been permitted by the introduction of the computer. As we have only a vague understanding of human intelligence, the potential of artificial intelligence is restricted to the application of programs with a limited number of logical rules. Its introduction into the medical world can be dated to the beginning of the 'seventies. A small number of these artificial intelligence systems have been constructed, generally acting as some kind of large 'memories', so-called expert systems. Within these systems the general and personal knowledge of experts (in their own discipline) has been stored and has now become available to everyone who is in need of an expert judgement. In a very limited number of places these systems are in use in clinical settings. They all suffer, of course, from a lack of logical structure and standardized nomenclature in medicine. We shall present a concise description of one of these systems.

The term 'artificial intelligence' is generally accepted to include those computer applications that involve symbolic inference rather than strictly numerical calculation. It is based on the hierarchical structured cognitive models as they have been created by investigators like Newell and Simon (1972), Kleinmuntz (1968), Wortman (1972, 1970) (see also Chapter III).

AI systems represent knowledge in the logical structure of the *if* (premise), *then* (action) syllogism, which is known as the production rule model. It is claimed that this model allows the coding of general and specific medical knowledge, module structures, explanation and checking. Some authors assume it to be too rigid (Spiegelhalter and Knill-Jones, 1984).

The inexactness of medical reasoning is viewed as one of the main stumbling blocks to the strict algorithmic structure of AI programs. Shortliffe and Buchanan (1979) have turned to 'confirmation theory' which is descended from the distinction of Carnap between two types of probability: 'degree of confirmation' (Spiegelhalter and Knill-Jones, 1984, Sadegh-Zadeh, 1974, Braithwaite, 1968) and 'relative frequency', which was incorporated and implemented in Mycin, one of the first AI programs. As inference rules to these probability estimates do not exist, one has again to rely on subjective estimations.

In one of the most sophisticated AI programs, CADUCEUS, the inference rules are largely based upon the introspection of one or more internists (McMullin, 1983). The contents part was derived and updated from medical literature (pathophysiological conferences, etc.). Unfortunately, because of its inductive inference rules, there is no automatic learning function built into the system. The crucial notion that the system employs is that of 'evoking strength' (ES), relating manifestations (M) to disorder/disease (D). The various possible diseases are organised into a hierarchy generated as information about each disease. Each disease corresponds to a node in the tree and is described by a set of atomic findings, each having two associated weights: an evoking strength ES and a frequency number (FN). ES depends on the likelihood that D and M in the pertinent population are causally related, estimated by the physician on an integer scale running from 5 (high) to 0 (low). ES, therefore, depends on the availability of alternatives to D as causal explanations of M. The strength with which M evokes D will depend on whether M was brought about by other causes D1, D2 ... Dn, which is the likelihood of M/D, (McMullin, 1983). Or, in other words, when one encounters manifestation M how seriously would one entertain the hypothesis of D? Such a question, however, is contents dependent (Blois, 1983).

When some manifestations in M accompanying D are not found in the presented illness pattern CADUCEUS uses a second measure to weigh the causal strength of M to D. This measure is called FN (frequency number), ranging from 5 (all) to 0 (none) which measures the frequency in the target population with which D is accompanied by M. If FN is 5, then the anomaly is serious. FN is based on frequency counts in medical records, not on estimated likelihood. An 'import number' (IN) weighs the clinical importance of each M to D, based on pathophysiological theories and knowledge. However, the physician does not consider each M separately and implicitly assign measures to it. He looks for large scale patterns of a familiar sort where the Ms are interrelated in a causal way. McMullin mentions two inadequacies of the system:

(a) the absence of patterning ability that would allow the recognition of common manifestation-clusters (Mu);

(b) the inability to stimulate the developmental aspect of diseases, the way they present over time.

In my opinion, Shortliffe (1979) hits the mark about AI systems when stating: 'They try to model their system on human cognition. The problem, of course, is that we must first learn how human cognition works'.

Alternative decision making models

'The classical theory is a theory of a man choosing among fixed and known alternatives, to each of which is attached known consequences. But when perception and cognition intervene between the decision-maker and his objective environment, this model no longer proves adequate. We need a description of the choice that recognizes that alternatives are not given but must be sought; and a description that takes into account the arduous task of determining what consequences will follow on each alternative' (Simon, 1959). It is this arduous task in particular which can raise several cognitive and emotional defenses.

'Decision-making is reducing uncertainty in a problem situation' (Slovic et al., 1977). A harassed decision maker confronted with a complicated task suffers a decline in cognitive functioning as a result of the anxiety generated by his awareness of the stressful situation. Considerable stress can be evoked in a decision maker merely by his trying to cope with the cognitive limits on his ability to work out a good solution to the problem in hand. Next to cognitive complexity, there are major sources of stress in decision making, including profound threats to the decision maker's social status and to his self-esteem that intensify decisional conflict (Janis and Mann, 1977). Every problem to be solved has a more or less mental impact on the decision maker.

Theoretical reflections on problem-solving invariably show us how different our concepts of thinking processes are from what actually seems to be the case when confronted with real troubles. The cognitive functioning is affected by psychological stress. The difference between the well-trained versus the non-trained individual is often striking. Well-trained people are often less subject to intellectual deliberation.

Stress and uncertainty are accompanying elements of decision-making and, have been, thus far, subject to little investigation. According to Einhorn and Hogarth (1978), our culture does not encourage explicit representation of uncertainty; it tends to promote confusion between certainty and belief. However, the relation between stress and decision-making is noteworthy. It involves several features in the choices and applications of various decision-making strategies.

When there is a high level of uncertainty the amount of information search declines. The problem solver spends less time on the initial examination of the problem and enters the information processing phase much quicker than in a less stressful situation. One can observe that subjective uncertainty is inversely related to time. The greater the uncertainty the less people perceive the studying of the problem as a fruitful enterprise which can lead to a solution (Driscoll and Lanzetta, 1965).

Each person (subconsciously) knows his level of uncertainty which marks the difference between intelligent decision-making and panic, between looking for solutions and complete confusion. One tends to avoid cues that can stimulate anxiety or other painful feelings. It may sometimes help a person avoid becoming completely demoralized.

Placed in real-life situations individuals certainly do not behave like a cool calculator but more like a reluctant decision maker beset by conflict, doubts and worry, who struggles with incongruous longings, antipathies, and loyalties, and who seeks belief by procrastinating rationalism, or by denying responsibility for his own choice (Janis and Mann, 1977). In real life, people are exposed to various sources of information that can evoke a considerable amount of emotion. As emotions are, in a way, also information items (to what extent we have no idea at all) people are inundated by information. When the degree of complexity of an issue exceeds the limits of cognitive abilities there is a marked decrease in the adequacy of information processing. Moreover, determining all the potentially favourable and unfavourable consequences of all feasible courses of action would require the decision maker to obtain so much information that impossible demands would be made on his resources and mental capabilities. A person's first concern, therefore, is to minimize the scale of the problem.

There are various ways in which this limitation can be effected, among which are:
- adapting to a more restricted level of aspiration (Satisficing, Simon);
- taking account of only a small number of – preferably related – options (Incrementalism, Lindblom);
- adjusting the problem to the solutions at hand (Garbage Can Model, Cohen, March and Olsen);
- stepwise elimination of the various options ('elimination-by-aspects' theory: Tversky);
- (or, 'No problem is so big that it can't be run away from': Peanuts).

According to Simon this minimizing process proceeds in the decisional task by imposing limitations on the scope of the search. It can be manifested as:
(1) when performance falls short of the level of aspiration, search behavior (particularly search for new alternatives of action) is reduced;
(2) at the same time, the level of aspiration begins to adjust itself downwards until goals reach levels that are practically attainable;
(3) if the mechanisms operate too slowly to adapt aspirations to performance, emotional behaviour – apathy or agression, for example – will replace rational adaptive behaviour.

The aspiration levels of people are, of course, arbitrary and subject to various circumstantial and personal influences. The aspiration level also has its impact on the scale of the subjectively estimated utilities. Adaptation of the aspiration levels, therefore, adjusts utilities in a similar direction.

Satisficing theory

In the viewpoint of Simon decision makers are adaptive; they adapt to the problem they are faced with. The decision maker is seen 'as a Satisficing animal whose problem-solving is based on search activity to meet certain aspiration levels rather than a maximizing animal whose problem-solving involves finding the best alternatives in terms of specified criteria' (Simon). The goal of the 'satisficing' person is 'to play it safe' by making decisions primarily on the basis of short term acceptability rather than by seeking a long term optimum. The strategy can be either finding an optimum solution in a simplified world, or finding satisfactory solutions in a realistic world.

Especially in repetitive situations, which are by definition simplified, this strategy may prove quite adequate. However, people tend to see repetitive situations when actually a new situation is presented. In our study, physicians assumed strong resemblances to cases they had recently met in practice, although the facts were quite different (apart from some initial data).

Satisficing is to settle for a barely 'acceptable' course of action that is better than the present state of affairs.

Incrementalism

In the incremental strategy, or the 'science of muddling through' (Lindblom,

1959), the attention of the decision maker is focused on only a few alternatives, which, preferably, are rather familiar to the decision maker. It is as if a physician, facing a patient complaining of headache, only concentrates on his having a 'cold' or 'stress', as he is most familiar with these ailments. The decision maker considers only a (very) limited range of alternatives with little attention to the consequences of these alternatives. For instance, the above-mentioned physician has on little evidence decided on a possible diagnosis of stress the possible consequences of which can be tested by prescribing a psychotropic drug of which he is only partially aware of its effects.

So, the decision maker is muddling through, succeeding in spite of in-competence or lack of method or planning. Lindblom saw this method espe-cially being applied in politics and large organizations, in which it fulfills the purpose of keeping the masses marginally content. But who is the physician who, honestly, will swear that he has never adopted this type of policy in order to keep the patient happy?

Incrementalism is a policy in which:

(1) ends and means are not viewed as distinct;
(2) the identification of values and goals are confounded;
(3) the policy maker subjectively views his policy as appropriate;
(4) the analysis of the task is drastically limited;
(5) the results of the policy are only compared to an older one ('the results were fine as I remembered from a similar previous case');
(6) there is a greater preoccupation with ills which are remediable rather than on seeking positive goals (after Sage, 1981). (For instance, physi-cians who are more preoccupied with treatment than with the establish-ment of diagnosis.)

Garbage can model

Although Cohen, March and Olsen (1975) set up the model as a model for organizational (university) decision-making, several features can be related to functions and decisions of persons in all sort of situations in daily life including clinical practice. It operates on the basis of simple trial-and-error procedures, the residue of learning from accidents of past experience, and pragmatic inventions of necessity. The model can best be exemplified by the following line: 'I have a solution, give me the problem that fits it'. This strategy can be exemplified to some degree by the generate-and-test strategy of Kleinmuntz and Kleinmuntz (1981) (see Chapter III).

The authors describe their model as a 'collection of choices looking for problems, issues and feelings looking for decision situations in which to be aired, solutions looking for issues to which they might be an answer, and decision-makers looking for work.'

In the medical world it can be translated as therapies looking for diagnoses, diagnoses in search of appropriate patient problems, biochemical tests looking for disease-entities still to be invented. It sounds ridiculous, but I am not so sure that these things do not come to pass in a harassed clinical practice. We have obtained indications from our study that at least treatment plans were confounded in the diagnostic reasoning process. From my own experience I can say that the availability of a remedy at least influenced the data-search. For instance, the availability of broad spectrum antibiotics diminished the need for extensive looking for bacterial classification in cases of bronchitis; indeed, the prescription of these drugs was time-saving, less cumbersome and less expensive for the patients. To enjoy an undisturbed weekend several physicians tend to prescribe more and more extensive combinations of antibiotics and chemotherapeutics to patients with urinary infections.

Solutions play a large part in this type of decision-making and problem-solving. The overall interest of physicians in remedies, treatment plans, and new drugs (described in Chapter I), can be seen as evidence for this approach. It is our impression that family physicians' behaviour must, at least partially, be understood within the context of the solution(s) they can offer the patient. The relation between the problem and the solution and their interactions has not thus far attracted much research attention. Some personal observations confirm this relationship. For instance, the way in which doctors restrict their search as soon as a possible solution enters their minds.

Within the model the solution is the key word, not the problem. The physician is then placed in the situation that there are various solutions available for one problem, and there can be several problems to cover one solution. The problem becomes a problem of what is the choice and what are the alternatives. Besides, the doctor knows that many problems resolve themselves spontaneously (wait and see). Sometimes an intercurrent problem interacts with the problem(s) already existing; this new problem is eagerly tackled in order to shift attention while hoping the other problems will evaporate. Sometimes patient and physician drag along for a long time; suddenly a remedy remotely connected to this complaint comes into view. This remedy will immediately be adopted by physician and patient as the solution to the (unresolved) problem.

Physicians are exposed to problems every day; problems which are not always resolvable; problems inherent to people and to circumstances. As most people know, one carries one's own problems, wherever one goes. Physicians are fully aware of this fact.

Conflict model

The last of the alternative decision models to be discussed is the conflict model of decision-making of Janis and Mann (1977). The authors base their model mainly on three issues:
   (1) the findings from experimental cognitive psychology about the limitations of the human mind for perceiving and processing information (which we discussed in Chapter III);
   (2) the tendency of people to avoid instituting a major shift in policy;
   (3) psychological stress as the concomitant factor in the decision-making process.

Although the existence of psychological stress and conservatism of actions is mentioned in the literature (Mason and Mitroff, 1973; Bariff and Lusk, 1977; Mischel, 1979; Albert, 1978), it has not received the attention it deserves. Especially in clinical practice where decisions can have far-reaching consequences this element can be of paramount importance. The competence of the doctor, the health and even the life of the patient can be at stake, families can be involved, and so on. The losses can easily dominate the gains, and, therefore, the level of conflict can rise in the extreme. Within this context the conflict model elucidates important features of clinical practice.

A 'decisional conflict' can be defined as 'the simultaneous opposing tendencies within the individual to accept and reject given courses of actions'.

As a psychological result of a decisional conflict the individual experiences feelings of hesitation, vacillation, feelings of uncertainty, signs of acute emotional stress. Depending on the magnitude of the conflict symptoms can even become of a physiological nature:, e.g., frequent micturition, frequent stools, headaches, etc.

A 'stressful' event is any change in the environment that typically induces a high degree of unpleasant emotion and affects normal patterns of information processing. Janis and Mann formulated five basic assumptions:

(1) the degree of stress generated by any decisional conflict is a direct function of the goal strivings that the decision maker expects to remain unsatisfied;
(2) when a person encounters new threats or opportunities that motivate him to consider a new course of action, the degree of decisional stress is a function of the degree to which he is committed to adhere to his present course of action;
(3) when decisional conflict is severe, loss of hope about finding a better solution than the least objectionable one will lead to defensive avoidance of the cues;
(4) in a severe decisional conflict, when threat cues are salient and the decision maker anticipates having insufficient time to find an adequate means of escaping serious losses, his level of stress remains extremely high and the likelihood increases that his dominant pattern of response will be hypervigilance. The persons's immediate memory span is reduced and his thinking becomes more simplistic;
(5) a moderate degree of stress induces a vigilant effort to scrutinize the alternative courses of action (..) and to work out a good solution.

From these assumptions 5 patterns of coping with stress are recognized by the authors.

(1) VIGILANCE: the individual is capable of effectiveness in an uncertain situation. It generally results in thorough information, search, unbiassed assimilation of new information, and effective planning.
(2) UNCONFLICTED INERTIA: if the oncoming disaster is of an unfamiliar nature, the person is likely to generate alternatives by searching his memory in an effort to remember similar threats encountered by himself or others in the past. An effective action will be taken if the

memorized alternative emerges into consciousness.
(3) UNCONFLICTED CHANGE TO A NEW COURSE OF ACTION: the person's aroused emotional state leads him to a defective coping behaviour if the danger materializes. His search for an effective action largely depends on this assessment of his own internal resources. If he cannot find an answer, the person will pessimistically give up searching for a better solution, despite being dissatisfied with the options that are open.
(4) DEFENSIVE AVOIDANCE: the subject will avoid cues that stimulate anxiety, uncertainty, stress or other painful feelings. The person becomes selectively inattentive to threat cues and avoids thinking about oncoming danger. Three forms of defensive avoidance are distinguished.
   – THE EVASIVE FORM: neglecting and ignoring elementary safety precautions, becoming fatalistically apathetic.
   – BUCK PASSING: depending upon someone else to make the decision. It may take the form of relying on outside agents of dubious reputation if they promise a less painful solution than the genuine expert who insists that the person himself must take responsibility.
   – BOLSTERING: ignoring available information and developing rationalizations which argue against the evidence of its potentially unsafe features. Typical examples of bolstering are to be found among certain types of cancer victims. Many of them ask no questions and selectively misperceive what their physicians are saying. They also develop rationalizations to convince themselves that their worries will be over after treatment.
(5) HYPERVIGILANCE: in its extreme form it is popularly referred to as 'panic'. The victim surmises that time is too short to make a (thorough) search for alternatives. He is overwhelmed by his emotions, unable to look for any effective action.
The three main stages of decision-making are relevant in all these five patterns of coping.
   (A) Appraising the challenge.
   (B) Thinking processes.
   (C) Making a decision.
We shall elaborate these steps in some detail
   (A) Before initiating a decision-making process people have to make up their mind whether to accept this challenge or not, i.e., 'motivation'. In the case of physicians there seems to be little choice, although in cases which are presumed to be of little importance the doctor sometimes denies his involvement. Most people prefer to avoid problems, especially the complicated ones. Politicians tend to focus on minor detials of complex, multi-faceted dilemmas, dilemmas which are so complex that really looking for solutions will create the possibility that one might burn one's fingers. Economists redirect the share-holders' attention from the firm's problems by starting a diversionary campaign. Judges

try to settle controversies by mutual agreement instead of solving the basic problem underlying the dispute.

(B) From the stage of motivation we enter the phase of deliberation. What kind of information do we search for? What is the price of more information? What is the amount of information related to the quality of the decision? What is the optimum amount we can process (information load)?

Most people begin to search their memory for similar cases in order to apply that course of action which was successful in previous cases, or they search for alternative courses of action which may fit the situation (compare garbage can model); or seek information from other people about the ways of coping. The information gathering is highly biased as people generally censor their intake of messages so as to protect their current beliefs and decisions from being attacked. Furthermore, people generally seek information that will support their prior attitudes and hypotheses. In clinical practice this can lead to funny situations: the physician as well as the patient are looking for supporting evidence to sustain their prior opinions. As they depend on each other's information, one can see a game of pleasing the other: doctors tune to patients and patients tune to the doctor in order to satisfy him (for being helpful in attending to their indisposition).

(C) Other psychological influences in making a decision are: regret and commitment. Regret means the difference between the reward actually obtained and the reward that could have been obtained with perfect foresight (actually with perfect hindsight) (Simon, 1959). In the case of an optimistic view people strive to maximize the reward; however, when expectations become adjusted at lower and lower levels, persons will strive to minimize the loss (see also prospect theory, Kahnemann and Tversky, 1978). In the psychological sphere it means that one is actually concerned about:
    − utilitarian losses for self;
    − utilitarian losses for significant others (e.g., peers, colleagues);
    − self-disapproval;
    − social disapproval.

Most doctors view themselves as reliable, competent, consistent, dependable, confidential, and generally gifted with considerable social feelings. Any loss of this self-image is seen as a serious loss and contributes to anticipatory regret, which in its turn can lead doctors to postpone decisions, and induce caution about committing oneself. His appraisal of the situation depends on:
    − the perception of having alternative choices; or
    − presuming immediate consequences to be involved; or
    − the decision as being of low social importance; or
    − conceiving impatience of significant others.

Any commitment which is assumed to be irreversible will jeopardize the making of a pertinent decision. Most people create some kind of possibility for retreat: 'do not stick out your neck, unless you are quite sure you can pull back your head'.

There are two aspects to commitment. Commitment is a good social function as it states: 'a promise is a promise', 'I can count on you'. It establishes social rules and social behaviour, it makes societies livable. Commitment allows for prediction of certain kinds of behaviour. It makes us rely on the advices of other people, like our physicians. Most people are not in a position to argue with the expert, so we have to rely on his judgement. His commitment makes us accept this judgement.

However, there is also another side. This side makes us stick to positions, chosen actions, ideologies and so on, despite increasing evidence for their opposite. It is very difficult to retrace one's steps without getting the stigma of being known as erratic and unstable. It is the keeping up of one's image as an effective, reliable person who can be decisive and who can keep his word. Many men experience great difficulty in admitting to having bought the wrong automobile; women in having bought the wrong dress, etc., physicians in admitting to having made a wrong diagnostic or therapeutic decision.

This effect is often abused by agents trying to draw a person into some kind of deal, mostly an unfavourable deal, intentionally or unintentionally. The intentionally deceptive agent employs a number of tricks to involve you in a deal which is mainly favourable to the agent himself. It is a process of emotional adaptation by agreeing upon some kind of unjustified rationalization that justifies to the person what he has done and then continues to draw him into actions with still some more involvement which is again justified and draws the person further and further in a direction which is certainly completely unwanted had the person known it before.

These types of commitment can be seen in the clinical domain. For instance, when a doctor has difficulty in persuading a patient to initiate a particular kind of treatment, he sometimes tries to persuade the family of this patient or other influential people from the neighbourhood of this patient, thereby trying to get a foot in the door. Patients sometimes try to get the doctor involved in some action he rejects in principal, but by social or other pressure is prepared to concede. Physicians expect the patient to commit themselves to the solution, the treatment action he prescribes. When the patient is averse to this commitment he is accused of non-compliance, which is socially and medically unacceptable.

Commitment is a strong force in the decision process: the higher the degree of commitment the higher the effects.

(1) The higher the degree of commitment the lower the probability that the decision maker will lightly dismiss the risks associated with changing to another alternative.

(2) The higher the degree of commitment the higher the probability that the decision maker is pessimistic about finding a course of action better than the current one.

(3) The higher the degree of commitment the lower the probability that any alternative to the original course of action will be selected (when the decision maker reaches the point of weighing the alternatives).

(4) The higher the degree of commitment the higher the probability that a

temporarily selected better course of action will survive a final questioning by the decision maker;

(5)   The higher the degree of commitment, the less likelihood that any given loss entailed by the decision will constitute an effective challenge.

The physician is committed to behave as rationally as possible within an environment of large cognitive burdens and a considerable amount of psychological stress. The physician has to strike a balance between these basic ingredients of clinical practice. How he must do it and how he can do it is a problem waiting for an answer. We presume that practising physicians will have to wait for a long, long time.

Summary

We discussed in this Chapter classical decision theory as the third branch of the tree of human thinking processes after thinking and problem-solving. As the literature on decision-making has piled up toweringly high we restricted the discussion to some basic principles of a number of theoretical models and their relation to real-life situations, especially with regard to the acting physician. As is the case in many sciences it is precisely here that differences of opinion appear and have given rise to manifold systems. These systems are meant to aid the physician in his clinical practice which deals with some difficult but mostly with a large number of routine cases.

Especially with regard to the latter facet we conclude that the most influential model, the rational decision maker model as designed by Von Neumann and Morgenstern and their successors, has failed in its mission. Its overall acceptance in the medical world is minimal in spite of all the optimistic statements its supporters. It also failed in its original mission to be an explanatory contribution to those parts of the human problem-solving processes in which man acts rationally in order to maximize his gains and minimize his costs (utilitarian theory).

We criticised several fundamental issues in this theory. These include utility and probability estimations, the conditions of independence, the problem of large numbers, Bayes' theorem, and the processing of information. None of these items can stand up to severe scientific analysis insofar as that is discernible from the literature. That, as Kassirer *et al.* (1987) remarks, is because 'almost none (of the papers) generate detailed technical discussion about the analytic methods used.' It is in their view part of the 'lack of self-criticism in the field'. We have to realize that 'clinical decision analysis remains more an art than a science' (Kassirer *et al.*, 1987). But this posture is to place the cart before the horse; it means that we shall replace an 'art-like' clinical reasoning which operates reasonably well according to the current standards of health care, with another 'art-like' process which has not even proven that it can reach these standards. Instead of creating an explanatory aid for physicians in order to upgrade their clinical judgements, decision theory diverts us from normal clinical methods in order to create a different kind of reasoning which seems at least as vulnerable as the 'normal' clinical reasoning which the information scientists consider to be inadequate.

It is my opinion that we shall have to retrace our steps, really observe what went wrong, and have the courage to depart from a route that obviously does not contribute to the assistance of the physician acting in his day-to-day clinical practice. A number of the alternative decision-making models like those of Simon, Lindblom, Janis and Mann, and Cohen, March and Olsen can, as explanatory models, assist in a redevelopment and a rediscovery of the original ideas about human decision-making.

Chapter V

Models and methods

> We impose our conceptions, our ideas and
> thoughts upon reality which creates prejudice.
> Prejudice precedes our view, our observation,
> and will determine what we shall see.
>
> B. Pascal

Introduction

When someone asks the doctor how he solves a problem or how he makes a decision, he usually gets some general answer which really says nothing about the actual process, or the doctor will, clearly amazed, ask, 'What do you mean?' The problem of the intellectual strategy, the way of reasoning, is not at the forefront of awareness in the medical world. Most physicians are completely indifferent to – even contemptuous of – clinical methodology. The general statement embraces the fact that every physician has his own pathways to diagnosis and treatment, and every investigation into this field must fail as a consequence of personal differences and the uniqueness of the patient-physician relationship. Most doctors are in fact unconscious of acting out a method. They rely on intuition and 'flair clinique' which is indeed a personally oriented approach unsuited for exploration.

But without any understanding of these processes we are still confronted by the questions posed in the Introduction, like, 'how do we know what we are doing?' and, 'how do we know that our actions are the most valid and reliable ones?'

In addition, another important question emerges: 'how do we teach future generations of doctors how to reason in problematic situations?' and 'how can we evaluate the effects of our solutions to the problems as presented by the patients?' How can we teach clinical medicine when we leave it to the students to deduce, to sense, the reasoning methods employed in clinical practice?

A small number of studies have been performed to understand and explain clinical methods. The growing interest during the last decades must, in our opinion, be attributed to the difficult and embarassing questions that have frequently been asked, and are still asked, by people engaged in the discipline of clinical decision analysis. However, an explanatory answer has not been provided. As we discussed in Chapter IV, clinical decision-making turned to the development of methods appropriate to its own approach, which might deviate from the methods that are actually used in clinical practice.

These latter methods have been the subject of a number of studies mainly from the psychological viewpoint. Though their contributions are valuable, in our opinion they missed the medical touch, the understanding of how the medical processes really go on. 'These studies have to be performed by people who really know what doctoring is' (Biörck, 1977).

This study is an attempt to approach the issue from the medical side. I am acquainted with clinical practice, I can understand the problems inherent in routine health care, I can speak the 'language' of doctors, and I have easy entry to physicians' offices. However, this pre-knowledge can easily create prejudice; it can blurr the vision; it can lead to observational errors. Models can help to restrict biases, because models make objective the ideas the investigator has in mind. Models can also highlight the criteria and landmarks of the processes involved so that objective testing is allowed for. Inherent to models is the possibility to be explanatory of a number of events which can be observed in the clinical process.

Following our theory we modeled the two ways of reasoning that are found to exist in inference processes: the deductive and the inductive. Adjusting these methods to the clinical situation, the models should be able to forecast particular outcomes inherent in these ways of reasoning (see Chapter II), given a particular input. Furthermore, the design of the model should neither be too detailed nor too general.

We defined three landmarks which are common to both models: hypotheses, symptoms, and the number of questions, and as a corollary, time. These landmarks can easily be traced in clinical processes and can also be measured with appropriate tools.

The most complex and comprehensive tool is the so-called 'paper patient' (Ridderikhoff, 1985). This instrument enabled us to provide standardized data as input into the physicians' problem-solving and decision-making task. It made it possible to locate and connect hypotheses to symptoms, to make unambiguous and mutual comparisons, and to simulate real-life situations.

The definition of levels of hypothesis-specification opened up the possibility of allocating hypotheses at particular places in a hierarchical system. Together with the symptom-coding system of the 'paper patient' particular lines of thought could be traced within the observed clinical processes. It furnished us with valuable data which brought this study to a conclusion.

Models in medical reasoning

When one asks a physician 'How do you make a medical diagnosis?' his explanation of the process might be as follows. 'First, I obtain the case facts from the patient's history, then I perform physical examination, and laboratory tests. Secondly, I evaluate the relative importance of the different signs and symptoms. Some of the data may be of first-order importance and other data of less importance. Thirdly, to make a differential diagnosis I list all the diseases which the specific case can reasonably resemble. Then I exclude one disease after another from the list until it becomes apparent what the case can be' (Ledley and Lusted, 1959). Evidently, it is a reasoning process of logical deduction and fits into the conception of the reasoning foundations as both those gentlemen described it in their fundamental and entertaining paper. On the basis of a scientific theory of diagnostics, and a firm and consistent conception of symptoms, signs and tests, valid, i.e., pertinent and relevant, hypotheses can be postulated which may cover the collected evidence. In order to discriminate between the hypotheses an analysis in the form of a series of argumentationsteps will be performed to reach a level at which each hypothesis will become testifiable, i.e., falsifiable in the light of the collected evidence. The hypothesis that can best stand the test can be chosen as the working diagnosis (it can never be the ultimate diagnosis, because, as we all know, in medicine and biology new evidence can always come forth and cast new light on the case). However, to my knowledge, this version of medical reasoning is hardly representative for physicians as a group, especially not in the world of family physicians.

Studies by Leaper *et al.* (1973) and Hull (1972) revealed a great variation in diagnostic pathways. They even question the existence of a common denominator in reasoning methods.

Evidently Einstein was right when he warned: 'If you want to find out anything from the professional worker about the methods they use, I advise you to stick as closely to one principle: don't listen to their words, fix your attention on their deeds.'

To get new incentives in medicine we need first to search for and then to analyse the individual work routines. The rationalization behind this approach is that physicians, either consciously or unconsciously, make similar judgements daily; they are faced more or less with the same problems; they all have practically equivalent therapeutic possibilities available; and they meet and understand each other wherever in the world on matters of problem-solving and practice-burdens. That means that physicians can recognize elements common to their processes, that they operate along rough guidelines distinctive of them all. It is our opinion that physicians have more in common than divides them. However, they view themselves differently from the way they really are. Usually they perceive themselves as they are pictured in public opinion and in literature. Pauker *et al.* (1976) picture the difference between the expert in practice and the expert as often pictured in literature or folklore. 'The epitome of the experienced physician in fiction is the detective who, through superior deductive powers and by sheer force of logic, organizes the facts at hand in a way that leads to a single, inevitable conclusion. By contrast, the real-world physician seems to rely much more heavily upon 'guessing', his initial hypothesis typically being based on precious little data'. These 'guesses' are apparently prompted by patterns of clinical findings or by specific complaints which bring to mind particular diseases. The physician then tries to demonstrate the correctness of his 'guesses' and moves to new hypotheses only if his initial impressions prove untenable. Apparently, judgements seem to be made to the extent to which the displayed features presented by the patient appear representative of the stereotype the physician has in mind. The more numerable and the more specific the stereotypes the physician has in mind the more he has a 'clinical view', 'clinical intuition', 'flair clinique'. But this theme only acknowledges the existence of pattern recognition as one of the elements in the diagnostic process, not its procedure.

From these approaches we can assume another process or processes different from the one described by Ledley and Lusted. Following our theory we predicted the other process to be an inductive one. We are convinced that most processes, though assumed to be idiosyncratic, can be allocated to the two methods of inference sketched above. We tried to organize these processes into formalized models.

Several recommendations have been made with regard to modelling the medical process (Pauker *et al.*, 1976; Gorry, 1974; Elstein *et al.*, 1972). The main requirement for a formalized model is that it must be intimately related to the actual system, the actual system which encompasses its structure and its behaviour. By structure we mean the totality of the interrelationships among its elements; the behaviour of the system is composed of the interactions between the system and its environment (see, e.g., Brunswik's Lens model, 1952). The aim of the model must be to 'represent' or to 'simulate' the hidden cognitive processes of the physician as he makes his judgements.

The use of models in studying medical problem-solving has been infrequent. The motivation for a model may come from several sources. For instance, a model may:

- isolate and illuminate certain relationships or properties of the modeled system and hence promote an improved understanding of that system;
- manipulation of the model is easier than real-life situations;
- experimentation and testing become less complicated.

Unfortunately, the potential advantages of modeling the clinical process are not generally recognized:

(a) many medical people seem to feel that a model of diagnosis must be complete, and hence so complex as to be unfeasible;
(b) the potential advantages of modeling as an activity are not generally recognized (Gorry, 1974).

A model, therefore, must indicate exactly what it is intended for: illuminating the highlights, the landmarks of a system. It has to elucidate the general outline because too much detail blurs the vision and causes one to miss the forest for the trees.

According to Pauker *et al.* (1976), the development of the model will require the efforts of physicians experienced in diagnosis. To a certain extent, the model makers also should consider concepts developed in other fields including cybernetics, cognitive theory, utility theory, and computer science.

To model the medical process, Elstein *et al.* (1972) recommend the following tasks:

(1) identify the intellectual strategies and tactics characteristic of clinical reasoning;
(2) generate a (psychological) theory to explain these features;
(3) relate this theory to current theories of thinking, human information processing, decision-making and problem-solving.

Styles of problem-solving and decision-making

When observing people solving a problem the impression arises that every-body operates in his own style, as a kind of personal trademark. Upon scrutinizing these processes, however, it appears that they have much more in common than divides them. The question is whether the common features can be classified into a general taxonomy. In our opinion, styles of problem-solving and decision-making can be arranged according to three categories.

(A) Personally induced.

(B) Problem oriented.

(C) Inferential approach.

(A) Several authors have tried to categorize and systematize the various problem-solving and decision-making processes by the personality structure of the actor. Mason and Mitroff (1973) suggest that varying psychological person-alities give rise to varying qualities of information gathering and evaluation. For the data acquisition side they define at both extremes: sensing-oriented types (preferring detailed, well-structured problems) and intuitive-oriented types (disliking routine tasks). For the information-evaluation side they define at the extremes: feeling-oriented individuals (relying on emotions, personal values, etc.) and thinking-oriented persons (relying on logical arguments). Obviously, there are several variations in between.

McKenny and Keen (1974) come to a similar organization of personalities. In the information gathering phase they recognize two types of personality: a preceptive person, focusing on patterns of information and looking for devia-tions from or conformities with their expectations; and receptive people, focusing on detail rather than on patterns. On the evaluation side there are also two types: a systematic actor, structuring problems in terms of some method, and intuitive people using the trial-and-error mode, relying on in-tuition and experience.

Bariff and Lusk (1977) distinguish abstract versus concrete (or systematic) reacting people in the information gathering phase of the process; and heuris-tic versus analytic at the evaluative stage.

It is beyond the scope of this book to discuss these and other types of personality classifications. In our opinion, these efforts cannot lead to a more definite explanation of problem-solving processes. These ideas are not only based on a broad and imprecise classification, but it also moves the explana-tion of the problem-solving process to an even more difficult problem: how to establish (unambiguously) a particular personality. Furthermore, these ideas focus on only one side of the process. In every problem-solving process two parties are involved, influencing each other in an often mysterious way. This influence can especially affect some characteristics of the personality of the problem solver. It is hardly realistic to disregard the opinions and attitudes of the other party. Even if one were to try to classify all people into a limited number of reacting types, even then the permutations of every imaginable possibility will lead to situations beyond our comprehension.

We can observe in each of these classes two types: an abstract-sensing-receptive personality and a concrete-preceptive-intuitive creature on the information-gathering side; and on the evaluative side we discover quite similar types of personality: thinking-systematic-analytic versus feeling-heuristic-intuitive. Disregarding the difference between the acquisition and the evaluative side of the problem-solving process (should there be any difference?), we are inclined to combine the characteristics of these personality types into the two prototypes of scientific reasoning: the logical, abstract thinking and the intuitive, concrete thinking. In this way the description of the personality characteristics as described by the various authors exactly into our description of the two ways of reasoning as we depicted in chapter II.

(B) Problem-orientation of the problem-solving process has been repeatedly mentioned in the literature (e.g., Pauker et al., 1976; Elstein et al., 1978; de Groot, 1961; Newell and Simon, 1972). The task governing the processes involved in problem-solving sounds a reasonable proposition. Janis and Mann (1977) suppose it to be impossible that new problems can be solved with old rules. Undoubtedly, every new problem as defined in the strict sense given in Chapter III, evolves new possibilities and asks for the creation of a 'new' problem space. But to ask people to develop new rules, time after time, is, in my opinion, asking too much. In mathematics a limited number of rules is applicable to a large number of problems. By combination and variation this limited number of rules can serve several goals. The problem space, as it is defined by Newell and Simon (1972), defines the pertinent knowledge and relevant rules apposite to the case at hand. However, what may be clear in mathematics (pertinent knowledge and relevant rules) is unclear in the clinical setting. As we discussed in Chapter I pertinent knowledge is usually personal knowledge, and relevant rules are wanting or at least unfamiliar to the problem-solver (see above). Within the clinical context problems seem to be approached by personally oriented methods creating personally oriented problem spaces. It means that problems cannot unambiguously be classified into a generally accepted system as one can in mathematics. When such a system is not available problem oriented explanations do not seem to fulfil our purpose of explaining the clinical process.

(C) We have chosen to adopt the inferential approach as decisive for modeling the medical process. As mentioned in the Introduction we have adopted the reasoning methods as they are used in medical practice as the prime source for our statement. We followed the Popperian line demarcating science from art by means of the two inferential processes: deductive and inductive. In our view, induction stands for the art-like conception of medicine, while, conversely, deduction stands for the scientific side. This thought has been further elaborated in Chapter II. It now serves for modeling both methods with particular respect to medical practice. The modeling has not only to deal with cognitive activities of a single judge or doctor but has to elicit the criteria by which a specific method can be recognized. The test of the model is not only how well it works as a representation of the state of the world, but also how well it predicts the inferential products of the judge

himself (Goldberg, 1968). If the model elucidates general principles of diagnostics, then it has both validity and value in teaching and decision-making.

The models

Models describe processes in gross features. The model delineates the landmarks within the process as they might be observed in the performance of the
task. These landmarks can be viewed as points of emphasis as they have
appeared in thought or have originated from observation or from literature. It
may be clear that not all features and characteristics can be included in the
model. The more we go into detail, the more we run the risk of emphasizing
the – personal – differences rather than the common characteristics.

The focus of this investigation should be the formulation of a 'general'
model of the medical process and its subsequent comparison with to 'real'
situations. The formal definition of what constitutes a model of either the
behaviour or structure of a given system is not an easy task. The key issue is the
elucidating of several features in the medical process in order to contribute to
the understanding of clinical reasoning.

Deductive model

The doctor who described his reasoning process to Ledley and Lusted gave an
excellent example of deductive reasoning. He brings the two main elements of
reasoning into contact. These two are: (i) if and only if the evidence covers the
hypothesis(es) and, vice versa, a testifiable case can be made, and (ii) by
narrowing down these hypotheses (from universal to specific) to a level at
which a singular test can be performed in order to verify or falsify the hypothesis (and thus all hypotheses in the hierarchy), is he able to judge the result (see
Chapter II).

It follows from the characteristics of the deductive reasoning that only one
hypothesis can be verified, or better, resist falsification. When two hypotheses
can explain the evidence as collected than there is no ampliative support for
either of the hypotheses: it is only tautological. So where more than one
hypothesis remains after the deductive inference process the doctor has to start
again from the beginning.

We can now depict the medical deductive inference process in the following
scheme in which the progression down the levels process is viewed as a series of
argumentation-steps (a term borrowed from Sadegh-Zadeh, 1974).

After the presentation of the patient's complaints and the subsequent data-
collection by the physician either by interviewing or by physical examination,
the acquired data have to be carefully analysed. As we pictured in Chapters I
and III the acquisition process as well as the reliability of the data can give rise
to profound and misleading errors. This phase of data analysis (and subsequent recording) seems to be of the utmost importance in the process. By
comparison and rearrangement of the data several hypotheses as configurations of symptoms and signs can come to mind. For instance, the hypothes-

THE DEDUCTIVE SCHEMA

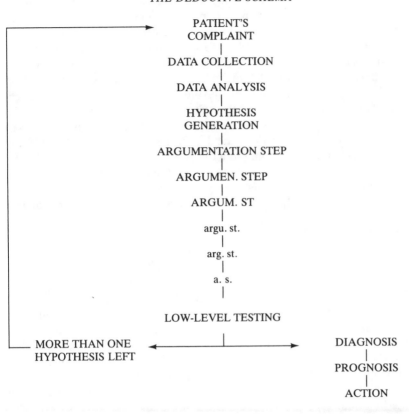

es may be: physical or mental, systematic or local, infectious or non-infectious, etc. The acquired data enables the physician to reduce those first hypotheses to a more specified level, like: physical→infectious→respiratory organ. A next argumentation step brings the doctor to the nearer specification of an infection of (one of) the lungs for which a number of symptoms and signs in his data-collection gives him sufficient evidence. Other symptoms and signs lead eventually to a specified hypothesis which can be tested by one or two proving instances, e.g., a bacteriological and a serological test. The ultimate testing verifies or falsifies the hypothesis. When the hypothesis is falsified the hierarchy of hypotheses falls down and the physician has to restart the process. In the case of verification the final hypothesis (= diagnosis) excludes other options open to the case and enables the doctor to proceed to appropriate action (treatment).

Inductive model

The next doctor is an inductive reasoning person. Asking him, 'how do you make a medical diagnosis?' we may get the following story.

D: First, when the patient tells me his complaints one or two ideas immedi-
     ately jump into my mind. Thanks to my experience I have quite a number
     of pictures in my mind. Some of them fit the presented complaints. Then
     it is my task to verify this idea, this hypothesis. So I ask a couple of
     questions looking for analogy with the picture in my mind. Sometimes the
     answers to my questions do not fit the predefined idea, so I have to drop
     the hypothesis. As a result of my interviewing, however, I have got
     several other ideas, so I can formulate a new hypothesis which again is
     verified with a couple of questions or examinations, and so on. Thanks to
     my experience most of the time I only need one round of verifying
     questioning in order to come to a diagnosis.

Q: So you go on questioning and examining the patient until the collected
     information perfectly covers your memorized picture of the disease?

D: No, not necessarily. It is a matter of similarity, not of complete congru-
     ence.

Q: But what about the other formulated hypotheses? In a way they also
     resembled your memorized pattern.

D: Yes, indeed. These hypotheses are not really refuted but serve as a
     collection of possibilities to which I can always return.

Q: But why should you prefer a second hypothesis to the first one? Does the
     second hypothesis encompass the first on the basis of broader evidence?

D: No. A hypothesis is a memorized picture as I have observed in practice
     more or less frequently. So hypotheses are rather specific. Each hypothe-
     sis, therefore, is tested for itself, and the more symptoms and signs that
     are congruent with the pattern I have in mind the more I am convinced
     that it is the correct diagnosis. The second hypothesis is not inferred from
     the first one.

Q: So you collect a number of hypotheses all of them with more or less the
     possibility of becoming a diagnosis. But how do you decide?

D: Well, at the end of the questioning and testing, (remember time is very
     important in our business), I reconsider all the collected hypotheses and
     choose the one that suits me most; the one that is the most attractive to
     me, which I intuitively feel the most probable one and of which I am most
     certain. That may not necessarily be the last generated hypothesis.

This picture of the reasoning method differs greatly from the first one.
Contrary to the linear and systematic method of deductive reasoning the
inductive method gives the impression of a vacillating or at the best a circular
strategy. It relies heavily on personal intuition and experience, and is typically
based on the attempts to determine whether alternatives are pleasant or
unpleasant, likeable or unlikeable, good or bad for individuals, or whether
they will satisfy the patient.

We shall summarize this method with the schema delineated by Medawar
(1969) for the inductive process.

   (1)   Early hypothesis generation based on analogous reasoning or (pattern)
         recognition. Analogies coming from strong memory patterns.
   (2)   Limitation of the observation, as the act of observation is governed by

the belief in the formulated hypothesis.

(3) Confusion of the formation and judging processes of the hypothesis.

(4) (Very) restricted possibilities to retrace the processes.

(5) Personal belief in the statement as arrived at by analogous reasoning from personal knowledge (as contrasted with general knowledge) makes rejection improbable.

(6) Final choice is made on the ground of 'satisficing': the hypothesis that minimally satisfies the personal standards of the decision maker; (see also Simon, 1959).

(7) Final choice is carried out by comparing the acquired hypotheses to each other.

(8) It sets no upper limit to the number of hypotheses we might propound to account for our observations. In real life the limits are set by our sense of idiocy or absurdity. In contrast with Medawar we assume 'time' to be a reasonable limit for the doctor in clinical practice.

For the medical reasoning process we have delineated the inductive method as follows.

THE INDUCTIVE SCHEMA

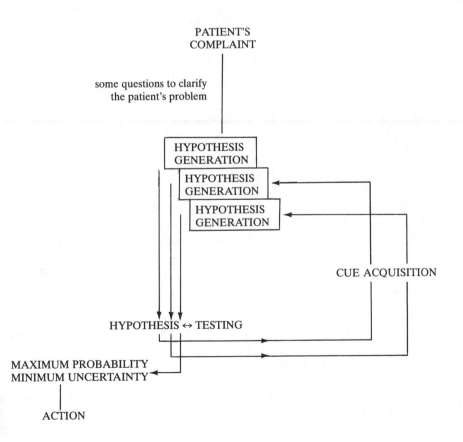

Hypotheses

Although the hypothesis as a concept is placed at the centre of each method as a major characteristic feature, we have to realize that the same name can cover different conceptions in the different reasoning methods. The hypothesis in the deductive process is clearly deduced from the acquired evidence. In its most elegant form the evidence covers the hypothesis in an exhaustive manner. All symptoms and signs can be explained by the hypothesis (diagnosis). A patient who complained about nausea and a vague pain in the middle of the abdomen, gradually descending to the right lower quadrant, and becoming worse, low fever, palpation tenderness on McBurney's point, positive rectal examination, elevated number of leucocytes might be diagnosed as having appendicitis as this diagnosis completely covers the symptoms and signs. This is exactly the way every student learns disease descriptions from his teacher and from a textbook. In strict logical terms we can denote:

$$C(h,e) = 1$$

or, the hypothesis 'h' is completely ($= 1$) confirmed (C) given evidence 'e'.

Unfortunately, nature still resists what doctors decide. This ideal situation is seldom (almost never) met in practice. In that case the reasoning has to take into account an alternative hypothesis also explanatory of most of the symptoms and signs, or in logical notation:

$$1 > C(h_1, e) > C(h_2, e) > 0$$

In this case we have to find a test which assigns a greater plausability to one hypothesis than to the other. We cannot prove beyond doubt that of the one with the greater plausibility is the definite one, but we accept it as a working hypothesis for the moment. We can say, the hypothesis is corroborated (confirmed).

In the inductive reasoning process we seem to deal with a different kind of hypothesis. Here there is no evidence to sustain the hypothesis as generated from the collected data. We can only accept this hypothesis if and only if we accept potential evidence (evidence from experiential knowledge) sustaining the hypothesis. It is small wonder that the hypothesis reflects this potential evidence. But even if we accept this inductive hypothesis as a deductive one, we also encounter in an abiguity. It is scarcely probable that evidence and hypothesis run in parallel. The evidence can transcend even the hypothesis:

$$C(h, e) > 1$$

which is incompatible with the theory. Even if the subjective probability is smaller than 1 we are in a quandary. How can we hold a particular hypothesis, that does not fit the acquired evidence, while being true to other hypotheses which likewise are incongruent with the evidence at hand? The formulated hypothesis can only be supported by some degree of belief.

The hypothesis in inductive reasoning is mainly the idea which the physician has in the mind. This idea is triggered by a small number of data so that it 'pops' into the mind. For instance, a small number of features makes us recognize a friend (almost) immediately; from the corner of an eye we can recognize a traffic situation perfectly and react accordingly. If we were to decompose this traffic situation into its elements, analyse these data, generate a (couple of) hypothesis(es), which we could subsequently test against the available evidence, we might eventually have found the solution but be on our way to the hospital. It is certainly not the way we have to face the routine matters and dangers of daily life. Our potential, unconscious, knowledge enables us to react quickly and spontaneously. However, the path of this reasoning, the track of our thinking processes in these cases, might be as hidden from the actor as it is from the investigator. Any review of the situation leads to rationalization; it may lead to 'telling more than you can know' (Nisbett and Wilson, 1977).

Subtypes of inductive reasoning

Within the inductive method we modeled three subtypes which might characterize the main methods employed by the various groups of physicians (family physicians and general internists). Landmarks to elicit these subtypes have to be found in our material. As a complicating factor the task environment of the two groups of physicians differs. The interaction of these two elements, strategies and task environments, could not be predicted but has to be empirically elucidated from the material. We defined three strategies: pattern-recognition, inductive-heuristic, and inductive-algorithmic.

PATTERN RECOGNITION

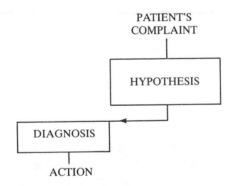

Pattern-recognition may be seen as the basic characteristic of the inductive model. It can be defined as the process of matching a patient symptom configuration with those configurations that the physician has memorized either from literature or through personal experience.

Those physicians who ask only a few questions beyond the presented complaint, take a decision and then design a treatment plan, are making use of the pattern-recognition strategy. It is the basic theme of the inductive method.

In most cases however, this elementary process does not lead to the goal of making a diagnosis or a plan of action. Second, third, etc., rounds are necessary in order to arrive at a satisfactory decision. The inductive-heuristic strategy is the iterative process on the basic theme. It makes use of clusters of symptoms and shortcuts in a quick cycling process. Data to the cycle come mainly from the testing of the inductive hypothesis, which, in fact, is a process of completing and confirming the pattern in mind. Any answer to a particular question of the physician can serve as a trigger to a new pattern. The term heuristic indicates that there is not a structured scheme according to which data are collected; the sequence of questions, examinations or tests is quite casual.

INDUCTIVE HEURISTIC

PATIENT'S
COMPLAINT

HYPOTHESIS
HYPOTHESIS
HYPOTHESIS
HYPOTHESIS

DIAGNOSIS

ACTION

stands for unstructured data-collection

The third variant of the inductive method is the inductive-algorithmic strategy. Fundamentally it is based on the same cycling process as the preceding variant. It differs from the former by its structured plan of strategy. In this study algorithmic has the meaning of:
- a structured plan of strategy by way of short runs of questions, examinations or tests in order to skim over the health or disease status of the patient and trying to avoid information gaps. The plan encompasses a structured questioning of each organ and behavioural system;
- the runs have a more or less characteristic form;
- the algorithm(s) are physician, not problem-oriented.

Landmarks in the models

From the description of the models we can now proceed to the delineation of the criteria for the various strategies.

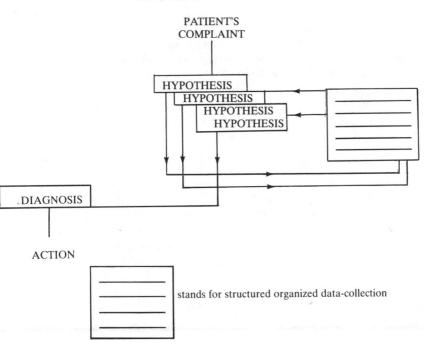

INDUCTIVE ALGORITHMIC

PATIENT'S
COMPLAINT

HYPOTHESIS

HYPOTHESIS

HYPOTHESIS

HYPOTHESIS

.DIAGNOSIS

ACTION

stands for structured organized data-collection

In their psychological model of diagnostic inquiry Elstein and colleagues (1978) used three features to account for medical diagnostic reasoning: information search units, cues (symptoms which may lead to a specific, diagnostic, hypothesis), and hypotheses. Cues and hypotheses were used as cross-cutting dimensions in a two-dimensional matrix according to which each simulation was structured. To determine the quality, the effectiveness and the efficiency of the problem-solving process, cues seen as related to a particular hypothesis were weighted according to a pre-established arrangement, based on expert judgements. According to McGaghie (1980) the selection of the variables seems partially to support partially the a priori thinking of Elstein *et al*.

To avoid interpretative variables we looked for objective criteria. Several landmarks within the medical process are submitted to subjective interpretation or can only be established with hindsight. Moreover, several of these features are interdependent. The weighing of a cue is a subjective interpretation relative to a specific hypothesis and to personal judgement. Redundancy can only be determined with hindsight. Whether an answer of a patient to a particular question will be positive or negative is quite coincidental as any arrangement of a patient case must come from real patients, not from the experimenter. When the patient's data did not fit the structure of the instrument, the instrument has to be re-arranged, and not vice versa. Whether an answer of the patient is taken as 'positive' (= any symptom or sign being deviant from normal function or form, and having medical significance to the physician), or 'negative', cannot be predicted. It is part of the arduous task of a physician that 'cues' have to be sought; they cannot be found by interpretation with hindsight. In the inductive reasoning 'positive' answers are very important; presenting them in advance is inducing the inductive type of reasoning.

Eventually, we decided on three basic features of analysis:
(1) hypotheses;
(2) symptoms;
(3) questions;
and as a corollary to create real situations,
(4) time.

(1) Hypotheses
With regard to the hypotheses three factors have to be distinguished.
– Their situation within the diagnostic process. Early generation is assumed to act as an incentive to early restriction of the problem space. It will certainly help the doctor to limit the strain on his cognitive abilities. On the other hand, it turns a blind eye to alternatives.
– Hierarchical nesting as a logical reasoning down the various patho-mental-physiological-anatomical levels distinguishable within the human body will provide a reasonable and at least a (re)traceable structure of the clinical reasoning process. Gaps in the reasoning process can easily be retraced by means of such a system of defined levels.
– Redundancy of hypotheses in a deductive reasoning process can only point to tautology, and is, therefore, incompatible with this type of reasoning. Evidence which is not explained by the hypothesis cannot be regarded as supernumerary. As we discussed above, evidence that transcends a final hypothesis is incompatible with deductive reasoning, but can be in complete harmony with inductive reasoning.

(2) Symptoms
For convenient reasons and because there is no essential difference between symptoms and signs (apart from their method of eliciting) we define 'symptom' as

'every functionally objective or subjective phenomenon which can be observed directly or indirectly and which is indicative of either an illness or condition of the patient'. (It also includes laboratory, X-ray reports, and similar types of data pertinent to a particular patient.)

As we discussed in Chapters I and III elements derived from or uttered by the patient must convey a particular clinical significance to the doctor before they can be acknowledged as medical datum. However, this 'significance' largely depends on the preconceptual opinion of the doctor (or the patient). When 'symptoms' presented in a (simulated) physician-patient encounter carry no meaning to either of them, there will be no real contact. In addition the symptoms have to be real, i.e., derived from real patients instead of being 'artificial' data from textbooks, etc. We had to be sure that the patient's meaning of his/her symptoms were unequivocally recorded. We did so by having the real patients interviewed and examined by a colleague (who was not involved in the study), and by checking relevant and pertinent items with their physicians (family physicians, consultants) as well as with family members and people concerned for the patient. When all the data were recorded in our predefined structure, called 'paper patient', we rechecked the items.

Secondly, we had to be sure that no differences of nomenclature between the physician and the 'paper patient' could disturb the results; unambiguous nomenclature was also needed for any form of comparison between the results of the participants-physicians' processes. We carefully selected all names of symptoms which might possibly have given rise to misinterpretation. From this idea evolved a completely new construction of symptoms and symptom-arrangements which we shall explain in the section on the 'paper patient'.

Thirdly, to convey clinical significance for the doctor means that the experimenter had to be able to relate the datum to an opinion of the doctor, in casu the hypothesis. Of course, it would be unrealistic to relate every symptom to a hypothesis, as the doctor might also have been 'looking around'. However, we hypothesized that at least 30% of all data could be connected to a hypothesis. If this limit could not be reached the structure would fail as a realistic tool.

Fourthly, the instrument should allow physicians to behave in a way that was as natural as possible. For instance, physicians are apt to jump from one class of symptoms to another, from social evidence to physical signs, from medical history to laboratory results, and so on. Any hindrance to this behaviour by the physician which was imposed by the instrument must be viewed as defect in the tool.

Fifthly, a question on the part of the doctor (which is sometimes difficult to understand) had to be connected to a particular symptom. When the question is too complex, the doctor has to decompose his question into simpler parts. Both partners, the doctor and the 'patient', have to be on terms with that part.

(3)   Questions

The physician's questions play a role at two different levels. First, they trace the process in its contents as well as in its sequence. The contents part may be quite clear. Every question is, we may suppose, aimed at eliciting a clinical datum (we shall leave aside all form of social talk notwithstanding its importance in the encounter). As we mentioned in Chapter I (on data recording) questions might bear a idiosyncratic mark. The combination with a – in the case of the experiment – standardized datum can therefore also define the question. It was the 'patient-physician-mediator's' task to elucidate those questions which could not immediately be connected to a particular item. In these instances doctors asked complicated questions containing a number of 'sub-questions'. For instance, 'Do you experience the stomach pain before or after the meals or before or after taking an aspirin?'. The patient not only has the duty to decompose the question, but also has to decide which question to answer. These complex questions were frequently met in our observations.

Secondly, questions give an indication about the sequence of events. When we talk about early hypothesis generation we mean that the generation took place after the acquisition of a rather small number of data. Time is relevant insofar as questions and time are closely interconnected; this is not always the case as we shall demonstrate in the next chapter. The relation between time and questions can also vary with the subtype that was employed. Preformulated series of questions (as in the inductive algorithmic method) are formulated more easily and quickly than questions which are personally induced reactions to the patient's answer.

(4)   Time
The criterion 'time' is related to the number of questions as well as to the totality of the process. The relationship between questions and time is a complex one. It differs per physician, per types of strategy, and with the kinds of problem. Some relationship cannot be denied, although its explanation asks for detailed research. For the present study the 'time - questions' relationship also has a bearing on the feasibility of the experiment. The arrangement of the procedure must allow the physician to ask the questions at a pace which fitted his habitual working pattern.

'Time' in relation to the totality of the process was divided into two sections: the time needed to arrive at a diagnosis; and the time needed to decide upon a therapy. Together these sections stand for the totality of the process, from the first presentation of the complaint to the conclusion of the process.

'Time' also served as a measure for comparison of the doctor's behaviour in the experiment versus the workup in real practice.

RECAPITULATION
HYPOTHESES   – situational position
                – hierarchy of levels
                – redundancy
SYMPTOMS   – standardization of meanings
                – real patients material
                – prestructured storage and retrieval device
                – connectability to physicians' hypotheses
                – unrestricted questioning through the data base
QUESTIONS   – contents tracing
                – sequence tracing
TIME   – pace of questioning
                – process time(s).

These landmarks have to be connected to the tools, the instruments, in order that the characteristic features of the various reasoning processes can be recognized.

Instruments

Two major instruments had to be developed. First, the creation of an instrument that could fulfil most of the requirements of the previously stated landmarks and criteria. It had to meet the unambiguous storage of real patients' events, an unequivocal and fast retrieval, permit a flexible pace of questioning, standard meanings for patient, physician and mediator, unrestricted access to all (categories of) data, and allow for the connection of a singular symptom to a singular hypothesis. This device was called the 'paper patient'.

The paper patient

A 'paper patient' can be described as a multipurpose device suitable for a number of applications such as:
- simulation in medical education;
- simulation for research purposes;
- data storage and retrieval system.

Basically, paper patients are case histories narrated in the time sequence of the real patient. These case histories are formally structured by their composer. The structure partly determines its use. The formally structured paper patients are mainly used in medical education for training and examination purposes. Examples of this type of simulation format are the modified essay question, a case history divided into several parts with a number of (multiple choice) questions at every interruption; and the widely used patient management problem (PMP) formats and its variants. These types do not allow the physician (or the student) to follow his own cognitive pathway. As these simulation formats act as a yardstick for the cognitive abilities of students only one fixed way leads to an optimal solution (the diagnosis or a treatment). Alternative pathways lead to suboptimal solutions and consequently to lower gradings. These types do not fulfil our requirements. Besides, displaying the written scenario can suggest questions, options or categories to the testee that otherwise might not cross his mind: the so-called 'cueing-problem' (McCarthy, 1966).

In actor simulation an actor, usually an interested layman, trained to simulate a patient, is provided by a detailed synopsis of a patient problem, i.e., the personal and medical history part. It allows the testee to follow his own pathways, and it avoids the cueing problem. Although seemingly preferable, there are a number of disadvantages, such as:
- limited contents: the more facts the actor has to remember, the more liable he is to confusion and to forgetting; the more omission, the more constraint in the use of actors in simulation;
- restraint in the construction: the more complicated the patient scenario the more mistakes can be made;
- restriction of the mode: generally actors are not able to simulate the elements of physical examination or deliver the data base for their biochemical or X-ray properties;

- shift in role content: the repeated interaction with various physicians can lead to shifts in the contents and emphases of the patient scenarios;
- limited use because of the availability of actors in various appointments;
- high cost: intensive training and the aforementioned restrictions account for high costs, because several actors have to be used to fulfil the demands of more elaborate projects.

Actor simulation is exemplified by the 'high-fidelity' simulation used by Elstein *et al.* (1978) in the first part of their study.

Eventually, we chose a mixed form: a verbal presentation of a written patient scenario. The patient's case history is recorded in a prestructured system (cards, books). The user asks questions verbally of a mediator as though he, the mediator, is the patient. The answers were provided by the meidator from the – written – system. The verbal mode was found to be most enjoyable and realistic, which is consistent with the findings of de Dombal *et al.* (1971). This mode allows the testee to follow his own cognitive pathways and grants various scoring possibilities according to the individual's workup.

Formating this type of 'paper patient' requires a number of conditions to be fulfilled. It requires a structure in which particularity can be transformed into a system that is general to all physicians. For the construction we need to know how data are identified, how they are selected, how many data are appropriate, how to test data, how to process data. It is essential to know the contents and structure of the medical process or the various medical processes.

(1) The contents: the data and symbols which compose the basis for diagnosis and therapeutical management. The various constraints on these elements have been discussed elsewhere.

(2) The structure: the rules, the laws and sequences binding the data to verifiable or refutable concepts of disease or health status of the patient.

Thus far, most simulation models are built on a number of assumptions. From the various thoughts expressed a number of wishes, conditions and criteria for a simulation model could be formulated.

(1) Case histories as obtained from medical records or composed by expert groups must be replaced by a patient's data base to a high degree devoid of value judgements.

(2) Data acquisition and storing must be uniform and unambiguous.

(3) Data must come from as many sources as possible: the patient, his relatives, physicians, nurses, social background, etc.

(4) Data storage must not be submitted to a predetermined processing mode.

(5) Data must be gathered by an independent collector from real situations.

(6) The data must easily and quickly be stored in the system (high production rate).

(7) Retrieval of the data by the testee must allow an individual workup through the case.

(8) No cueing is allowed.

(9) Preferably the 'patient' is addressed verbally by the candidate. This means the use of a mediator between candidate and 'paper patient'.

(10) The mediator must be a trained person acquainted with medical jargon and be able to handle a large number of scenarios (cost aspect) without influencing the candidate.

(11) The system, including the mediator, must allow for a realistic provision of answers in a given time (number of questions per minute).

(12) The simulation must approximate to the setting and time constraints of the routine day-to-day professional activities of the physician.

(13) The scoring must be based on what really happens in practice.

(14) The scoring variables and their weights must be founded on a reliable and verifiable medical data base.

(15) The simulation must meet the qualities of validity and reliability (Ridderikhoff, 1985).

One of the bottlenecks in existing devices is the discrepancy between the available data and the number of options that could be handled by a candidate. According to Pauker *et al.* (1976) the estimated total number of facts in general internal medicine and its subspecialties (nephrology, cardiology, hematology) is about two million facts as the core body of information in this specialty. For general family practice this number can be doubled, even tripled or more. There seems to be no way of bringing these numbers down to a manageable format.

However, it crossed my mind that thus far simulations were adapted to medicine and not vice versa. But trying to inflict a more or less consistent system upon a rather unsystematic and huge body of data is likely to fail. The only possibility, seemed to me, was to systematize the medical data. It was of these thoughts that model originated. The system is based on the elementary attributes of medicine: symptoms and signs. Within this concept we face two problems:

– overcoming a huge number of facts; and
– having these facts standardized in an unambiguous way.

Upon studying various medical textbooks it occurred to me that several symptoms were mentioned more than once dependent upon the context in which they were used. They appeared in different forms and different settings depending on their causal relationships to each other or to the disease to which they can be attributed. Various names could cover the same meaning, different meanings could hide under one name.

The symptom pain, for example, was mentioned four, five, six or more times for one and the same disease, describing various states like: localisation, onset, irradiation, etc. It seemed that the entity 'symptom' is not the basic element in medicine. Russell and later Wittgenstein have proposed that the world might be susceptible to description in terms of (atomic) statements, 'propositions so primitive that they require no further explanation' (Scriven, 1979). In the same sense Blois (1983) advocated a 'downward analysis': from high levels corresponding to humans, to low levels corresponding to molecules and atoms. Crucial to the reduction of the amount of symptoms, therefore, is the re-

striction of the descriptions to mere observation (leaving out causal relationships, inferences, or interpretations) and the finding of common denominators
for equal reactions of the body or mind, functional or pathophysiological. A
second objective was to create a set of attributes describing all the various
aspects of a symptom; a set of attributes which gives a symptom its specific
significance. This set should preferably be pertinent and uniform to most of the
symptoms.

The human body has only a limited pattern of reactions to illness provoking
conditions, substances or infections. This notion has several implications. By
renaming similar symptoms their number can be reduced. Stimulation of the
mucous membranes, for example, gives rise to discharge whatever the localisation may be. The aspects of the discharge are equal for all localisations: its
character, colour, time of onset, course, etc. When discharge is a typical
functional reaction of the organism there is a strong motive to specify it a
symptom as such. The symptom 'swelling' cannot be differentiated from
benign or malign tumors without causal interpretation by the physician. The
symptom 'pain' can be fully described by a number of aspects, like: localisation, character, irradiation, intensity, seizures, relapses. Inferences, predictions or causal suggestions in the early phases of the diagnostic process can
often lead to confusion and erroneous ways of reasoning. Atomization of the
symptoms in medical history leads to an almost uniform set of aspects. They
can be listed as follows (in parentheses some aspects that can vary according to
the symptom to which they pertain):

- localisation
- character
- intensity
- irradiation (spreading)
- (colour)
- (odour)
- way of onset
- time of onset
- preceded by
- course of localisation
- course of character
- course of intensity
- course of irradiation / and/or spreading
- (course of colour)
- (course of odour)
- (seizures)
- (duration of seizures)
- (distribution of seizures)
- relapses
- combination with other symptoms
- combination with a body function
- worsened by
- improved by
- ahead of

For the symptoms of the physical examination a slightly different set of symptom-aspects was created. Within the framework of a particular organ system it was possible to create a nearly uniform set of aspects. Congruencies across the various types of physical examination were formulated. It will be exemplified by the symptom (Mal)Form(ation) = the description of the Form/Shape and its deviations from existing organs or body structures.

INSPECTION	PALPATION
– localisation	– localisation
– circumference	– circumference
– shape	– shape
– circumscription	– circumscription
– singular/multiple	– singular/multiple
– number	– number
– (im)mobility	– (im)mobility
– symmetry	– symmetry
– enlargement/reduction	– enlargement/reduction
– protrusion	– protrusion
	– pain on pressure
– ballottement	– ballottement

Also laboratory and roentgenological data were easily arranged under a limited number of headings, each split up into a limited number of elements. The same can be said for drugs, medical actions, etc.

Furthermore, a strict category of the symptoms was introduced, five classes for the diagnostic part, and two for the therapy part. These classes are:

(1) patient's personal, social, mental and environmental background; containing data about age, sex, marital state, education, occupation, finance, etc.;

(2) patient's past medical history, with items like: former diseases, operations, allergies, immunisations, child birth, etc. This class also includes surveillance programmes, mobility and activity scales, presently used drugs, etc.

These two classes combined can be described by 52 various symptoms, each symptom accompanied by approximately 15 aspects.

(3) Patient's medical history: the class of verbally communicated symptoms. This class is fully described by 68 different symptoms, each symptom accompanied by approximately 20 aspects.

(4) Patient's physical examination. Traditionally this class is divided into four subclasses: inspection, percussion, auscultation and palpation, to which, for practical reasons, is added a subclass for instrumentally obtained and observed symptoms such as: temperature, blood pressure, ECG, fundoscopy, etc. This class contains 141 separate symptoms, each symptom accompanied by approximately 15 aspects.

(5) Patient's laboratory tests, including data from roentgenological, bacteriological, pathological departments, containing 55 symptoms, each symptom accompanied by approximately 12 aspects.

Each symptom and symptom-aspect was coded according to the following attributes:
- positive/negative, depending on being deviation from normal health.
- class (of the paper patient) (upper case letters).
- organ system(s) (lower case letters).
- a figure for the symptom (1–500).
- a supplementary figure for the symptom-aspect (1–30).

The complaint 'pain in the neck' furnishes the code:

   + *D* bg 10.03.

The two classes for therapy are:
   (6) description of all possible actions a physician can take in therapeutic management and treatment; also including the description of referral destinations and types of consultation. This class contains 58 entries with approximately seven items each;
   (7) a detailed list of drugs classified according to their generic names; fysiotherapeutic, ergotherapeutic, and psychotherapeutic treatments and a not exhaustive list of alternative drugs and treatments. This class contains 97 entries with approximately 20 items each.

The total number of items in the 'paper patient' is approximately 7000.

Case histories for the investigation

For the research project nine real case histories were stored in the system. Each case history contained approximately 350 items deviating from normal health. These 3000 items could be stored for over 99%. This favourable result was checked by means of an independent test with 42 audio/video registered routine patient-physician encounters of independent family physicians. Two co-workers independently entered the registered data into the system. The result was the same: an average of 99%.

The described format is standard for all kinds of diseases with the exception – thus far – of psychiatric diseases. For each patient scenario a standard construction is used to which the patient's data are added. Computerizing the system is easily accomplished.

It takes two days to construct a 'paper patient' if all the material is collected. This material was acquired by thoroughly interviewing the patients, his or her relatives, family physicians, consulting specialists, nurses, social workers, etc.

The choice for the nine cases was based on:
- prevalence rates;
- age categories;
- sex;
- covering most organ systems.

Excluded from the selection were:
- rare diseases (very low prevalence rates);
- age categories. Children were excluded because of possible difficulties in taking the medical history directly from the patient. Elderly people were

excluded because of the possibility of multipathology;
– psychiatric diseases and disorders.
We have chosen the following categories:
(1) 20–30 years : man   : high prevalence;
             woman : high prevalence;
(2) 30–40 years : man   : middle ranking prevalence;
             woman : low prevalence;
(3) 40–50 years : man   : high prevalence;
             woman : middle ranking prevalence;
(4) 50–60 years : man   : high prevalence;
             woman : low prevalence.

The prevalence rates are all derived from a special epidemiological study of the epidemiological department of the Erasmus University, Rotterdam.

The choice of the various organ systems was made according to preliminary results from a classification project among family physicians in Rotterdam (Lamberts, 1982). These systems are:
Blood;
Circulatory tract;
Central Nervous System;
Dermatological tract;
Digestive tract;
Endocrinological tract;
Musculoskeleton tract;
Respiratory tract;
Urogenital tract;
From these criteria emerged the following sample of 'patients':
(1) Woman, 19 years, with hypochromic anemia;
(2) Man, 21 years, with atopic eczema;
(3) Woman, 31 years, with extra-uterine pregnancy;
(4) Man, 34 years, with asthmatic bronchitis/(chronic non-specific lung disease);
(5) Woman, 43 years, with gall-stones;
(6) Man, 41 years, with sciatica;
(7) Woman, 53 years, with hyperthyreoidism;
(8) Man, 57 years, with myocardial infarction;
(9) Woman, 47 years, with diabetes mellitus.
This last 'patient' was used as an instructive example for introducing the procedure to the participant-physician. The patients were included according to the (sometimes preliminary) diagnoses of their family physicians, who in the Netherlands constitute the first and only means of entry into the health care system.

Hypotheses and symptoms

Some remarks are required on the allocation of symptoms to the hypotheses. Symptoms (and their aspects) can be marks leading to hypotheses and particular items in the physician's reasoning process. Symptoms can be seen as the main data which can trace the diagnostic process. However, symptoms can indicate several diseases (and hypotheses), and symptoms can have various meanings in relation to different diseases or organ systems. It requires a standard symptom categorization in order to trace and retrace some aspects in the medical process. The application of a (re)tracing method demands:

    (a) that symptoms have to be recognized and coded in 'atomic' states; (atomic meaning: the lowest level of abstraction of unique patient signs on which standardization can take place);

    (b) that coding cannot be allocated to the physician's questions but to the 'atomic' symptoms (symptom-aspects) themselves.

For our purposes it seemed natural to code symptoms and hypotheses according to the various organ systems, being the level at which a non-committal allocation can be ascertained. Generally, hypotheses and most symptoms refer to only one or two organ systems. Those symptoms covering a larger domain are coded in conformity with all pertinent organ systems. (The term 'organ system' must be viewed in a broad sense.) The coding refers to the organ systems mentioned above (for scoring hypotheses of the mental diseases tract, this tract was added only for scoring possibilities).

The method of allocating a symptom to a hypothesis operates as follows: suppose that a hypothesis is generated referring to an organ system 'A'; the 'testing' symptoms (as related to the physician's pertinent questions) can be traced as related (HRS[1]) when coded for the same organ system. When the symptom's particular organ system code does not harmonize with the system code of the generated hypothesis, two possibilities can be distinguished. Either the symptom belongs to a non-committal search behaviour, and is unrelated to a particular hypothesis (NHRS[2]), or the symptom is related to a forthcoming hypothesis, a hypothesis pre-related symptom (HPS[3]). In the latter case the code of the following hypothesis, e.g., 'H', reflects the code of the symptom, which in that case can be allocated to the second round, etc. The cycling process can easily be traced from this procedure.

Two conditions were incorporated into the design:

    (1) the symptoms must unequivocally be recognized across situations; and

    (2) the symptom-coding must be in harmony with the coding of the hypotheses.

When these two conditions could not be fulfilled, the symptoms could no longer be viewed as tracers in the medical problem-solving process, which implied the failure of the system. The varying meanings of symptoms and signs, the non-uniformity of disease concepts, the ever-changing variations in the framing of questions by the physicians for particular symptoms, and the transient symptom-disease relationships during the course of an illness could only be marshalled when these data could be standardized and unambiguously

---

[1] Hypothesis Related Symptom.

[2] Non-Hypothesis Related Symptom.

[3] Hypothesis Pre-related Symptom.

allocated to that particular focus of attention in the physician's thought process: the hypothesis. Fortunately, it worked out.

Hypotheses levels

An unambiguous hypotheses-level recognition device was needed in our experiment. Several authors have recognized the importance of the definition of hypotheses-levels. None of the descriptions permitted an independent judgement across the various patient problems.

We developed a five-level physiomorphologic structure based on 'systems view of illness and disease' (Engel, 1980). This multilevel general systems model ranges in 14 steps from Biosphere to subatomic particles. Within this model five levels within the human sphere can be distinguished: person, mental system, organ system, tissues and cells. From this conception the following model was constructed.

Level I. Human being
Hypotheses referring to global descriptions comprising the total human being will be included within this category. It refers to descriptions like ill/not ill, mental/somatic, serious/not serious condition, etc.

Level II. Multiorganic formulation
Hypotheses within this class refer to pathophysiological states comprising more than one organ system. It includes diseases of body systems or body parts. The class can be typified by examples like: unspecified infectious diseases, unspecified neoplasmata, unspecified ailments of body parts ('something in the chest', 'abdominal pain').

Level III. Organ system
This class follows the normal medical distinction of organ systems. For instance, respiratory tract, digestive tract, musculoskeleton tract. All hypotheses referring to a certain organ system without further specification of the illness are included in this class.

Level IV. Organ
This class refers to specified organs and tissue-entities. It includes the nearest explanation to the specified disease entity. Hypotheses nominating the specific organ or tissue-entity are included. It can be typified as: gall-bladder disease, anaemia, eczema, etc.

Level V. Cellular
This class describes a specified bio-pathological state. It refers to all specific diseases generally described in medical textbooks. The hypothesis provides an exact circumscription of the lesion and its cause. For instance, duodenal ulcer, hyperthyreoidism, acute glomerulo-nephritis, myocardial infarction.

In a preliminary study the system was tested. Two independent judges classified 57 hypotheses according to the system. All hypotheses could be placed within a class; the inter-judge variability scored less than 5%. In the actual investigation general agreement could be reached for all 745 hypotheses. We judged the system fair enough to recognize a hierarchical structure of hypotheses.

Some minor devices had to be provided for. Probability estimations could play a role in clinical decision-making; a device for noting down these estimations had to be provided. Considering various alternatives we opted for the Euclidean method: placing points on a straight line delineating estimations between 0 and 1 (0 and 100%). Distances could be easily translated to preferences (see Chapter IV) and the method was easily adopted by the physicians. We supplied them with a form on which they could note down their formulated hypothesis and simultaneously give their estimation (prior probability) on one of the lines directly connected to the line for the hypothesis. Every hypothesis line faced three lines for estimations: one for the prior probability, one for cue-adjustment, and one for the posterior probability. Extra lines were provided for a manifold of cue-adjustments every time the physician felt an inclination towards revaluation of his probability-estimate. Only the first and the third line were used, although physicians were encouraged to use the other lines.

In the same way a number of lines were provided in order to estimate the personal feeling of (un)certainty about the course and the outcome of the process. The physicians were urged to assess their feelings every two minutes.

The completeness and the spontaneous way in which the physicians performed these tasks during the workup gave the strong impression of a sincere and natural expression of their feelings and their estimations.

Besides these forms the doctor was provided with his habitual papers, forms and prescriptions. For instance, the prescriptions were written out on the regular forms, the referral letters to consultants were written on the usual papers, etc.

Observational methods

Various methods have been described to study thinking processes. The implicitness of the subject forces investigators to make a selection of aspects or to choose from among types of research models. As sketched before, mainly two types of models can be distinguished:
  (1) prescriptive studies, which make use of a formal theory of how decisions ought to be made. Their aim is to build or to rebuild strategies according to which the medical process, the diagnostic as well as the therapeutic part, can be shaped or reshaped into an – easily – manageable structure which allows improved performance and productivity of this process;
  (2) descriptive studies which attempt to describe how human judgements

are actually made, including circumstantial and situational factors which influence judgements. Descriptive studies involve the problem solver's task environment.

Descriptive studies try to understand who the doctor is, what he is doing, how he functions and what his effectiveness as an information processor is. In other words, we refer to studies that try to understand all the medical actions which are laid down in the physician's professional duties and responsibilities. Surprisingly little research has been done so far on these professional activities. Notwithstanding a growing interest in this field, a number of methodological limitations seem to inhibit further investigations. Some of these limitations have been mentioned before including:
- the complexity of the medical system;
- the absence of a uniform, unambiguous medical classification system, and also
- the difficulty of observation in a patient-physician encounter. This encounter encompasses two systems, the patient's and the physician's. From this the main problem arises, because studying the functioning of the physician means observing these two systems which, at the same time, influence each other in a special, implicit way. It is like focusing on a certain point on a turning wheel while sitting on another wheel rotating in an opposite direction. One observes flashes only partly recognisable.

To gain a deeper insight into the working methods of physicians there are three principal methods of investigation which can be employed;
- observation;
- introspection; and
- simulation.

The observational methods seem to be the track with the highest validity. But they meet some major obstacles, such as:
  (a) the influence of observation on the doctor-patient encounter. The very fact of being observed may alter the nature of the situation which is being observed and documented (Leaper et al., 1973). Although both partners judge this influence to be of minor importance nevertheless we do not know its magnitude;
  (b) the complexity of the process. If one does not exactly know what to look for, one tends to a superficial selection of observations not only subject to the observer's variation but also to confusion. Confusion may arise as the process consists of qualities and elements of various specialties and disciplines;
  (c) the two-systems mode of the physician-patient encounter;
  (d) the ethical issue: guarantees of the patient's privacy and the physician's confidentiality cannot be maintained (Ridderikhoff, 1985).

Apart from this direct observational way indirect observation can be employed. Three methods can be identified:
- medical records survey;
- interviewing;
- questionnaires.

Medical record surveys can elicit a number of aspects in a broad perspective. The study of Noren *et al.* (1980) gives details about referral patterns, duration of visits, use of physician time, extent of diagnostic effects, efforts at patient education, and provision of personal advice or emotional support in a comparative study of 610 family practitioners and 347 specialists in internal medicine. For gaining insight into the medical problem-solving process this type of observational research is unrewarding.

Generally, medical records do not represent the most completely documented information source. The physician takes down only a limited number of mostly positively directed facts and aspects which are of special interest to him and the particular case. This is an unacceptable selection which does not allow one to draw special or general conclusions. The attempts to standardize medical recording (e.g., problem oriented medical record (Weed, 1970)) have failed to overcome a number of these problems. The strategies of interviewing and questionnaires fall mainly in the domain of introspection.

Introspection focuses on one of the two persons in the patient-physician encounter. It is based on – mostly retrospective – interviewing of the individual and verbal reports of the preceding problem-solving task. Several studies in the medical field have been reported among which are the famous studies by Kleinmuntz (1968), and Wortman (1972). However, several psychologists question the validity of these approaches. Nisbett and Wilson (1977) found that subjects, when asked about the answer they gave, to report on their memory of specific events, 'theorize' about their processes. Nisbett and Wilson came to three major conclusions:

(1) people often cannot report accurately on the effects of particular stimuli on higher order, inference-based responses. They sometimes deny an inferential process of any kind. The accuracy of subjective reports is too poor to produce generally correct or reliable reports;

(2) when reporting on the effects of stimuli, people may not examine a memory of the cognitive processes that operated on the stimuli; instead, they base their reports on implicit, *a priori* theories about the causal connection between stimulus and response;

(3) even if the reports are correct, this does not mean that the instances of correct reporting are due to direct introspective awareness.

Unfortunately, most studies reviewed provide little data as to what information is heeded during the thought processes. In a number of investigations the subjects were forced to infer rather than to remember their mental processes. Modern psychology has been vague about the use that can be made of these verbal reports. It may be clear that questions like: 'How do you do these tasks?' produce different reports from more precise questions. The former question implicitly requests a general, rather than a specific, interpretation of how the individual was performing the task in question. In these cases the subject may be drawing on prior information such as general knowledge on how one ought to do such tasks, to generate a verbal report describing a general procedure or strategy. They base their reports on implicit, *a priori* theories about the causal connection between the question and the response.

They cannot report on the cognitive processes which mediate between question and response because 'we may have no direct access to higher order mental processes such as those involved in evaluation, judgement, problem-solving, and the initiation of behaviour' (Neisser, 1967). 'It is the result of thinking, not the process of thinking, that appears spontaneously in consciousness' (Miller, 1962). Apparently, introspection is not a faithful instrument for revealing thought processes nor does it contribute to the accuracy of the reported verbalizations. However, Ericsson and Simon (1980) found that when people articulate information directly, verbalization will not change the course and structure of the cognitive processes. In contrast with retrospective verbalizations concurrent verbalization leads to more accurate reports on thought processes. What is remembered, and how well, will generally depend critically on the interval between past event and the moment of recall. Ericsson and Simon found that under certain conditions concurrent (immediately noted down) verbalization does not affect essentially the processes under study nor does it affect the speed of performance. When the time gap between verbalization and the attending instance widens, people have to rely more and more on memory. As we have discussed above, memory retrieval is fallible and may sometimes lead to accessing other related, though inappropriate, information. This may not be a matter of forgetting but of recoding of the information. The recoding process is performed on basis of the *a priori* thinking and conceptions of the subject. Any outcome of a mental process which is related to some recoding is directly associated with the *a priori* thinking. As long as the information resides in STM the information can be reported without bias. Ericsson and Simon, therefore, assume that only information in focal attention can be verbalized.

Kassirer and Gorry (1978) question the role of 'stimulated recall' in the Elstein *et.al.* study. Elstein and colleagues asked the physician-subjects about their previous thought processes while they watched videotapes of their earlier encounters with the simulated patient. Kassirer and Gorry think it possible that this retrospective verbalization may function in a way that would suggest hypotheses that might not have been evident from the presented data.

Retrospective accounts leave much more opportunity for the subject to mix current knowledge with past knowledge, making reliable inference from the protocol difficult. All theorizing about the causes and consequences of the subject's knowledge state is carried out and validated by the experimentee, not by the subject (Newell and Simon, (1972). We believe that an experimental design that relies heavily on retrospective observation is potentially flawed (Palva, 1974).

Simulation of the medical process encompasses two persons, the patient and the physician. Studying the doctor automatically includes a 'fixed' patient. A 'fixed' patient can only be a simulated patient, because real patients are never identical in different situations, different times and with different physicians. It also includes:

- different interpretations upon identical information;
- different framing of queries;

– misleading answers;
– changing symptoms and signs;
– varying kinds of questions asked, and
– differing sequences of questions (Gill *et al.*, 1973).

The simulated patient can present exactly the same clinical problem and the same clinical attributes to many different examining physicians. The variable has to be the physician, not the patient (Barrows and Bennet, 1972).

Generally speaking, there are three possibilities for patient simulation:
(1) 'actor' simulation;
(2) written simulations, with or without the intervention of a simulator;
(3) computerized simulations, with screen display and data storage.

Each of these items has its advantages and disadvantages.

Simulation procedure

The simulation procedure of the present study can be described as follows. After an appointment has been made, the research team consisting of a family physician (the simulator) and a technician set up the scenery of audio and video-recording apparatus in the physician's own consulting room.

Meanwhile the physician participant was instructed in two ways: first, he received printed instruction material outlining some of the items of the forth-coming procedure; secondly, the simulator instructed the physician verbally in detail and answered any questions which may have arisen in the candidate's mind. Meanwhile, the technical part was completed and the procedure was continued by 'doing' the instruction paper patient. All together, this in-struction and the set-up of the technical equipment took 20 minutes on average. In all cases it satisfied the instructional requirements.

The scenerio was arranged in the way the physician was accustomed to. It means that the physician was seated in his ordinary place and the simulator in the place intended for the patient. The videocamera (and the student) was situated at an angle which enabled the physician, his desk, his writing and a digital clock to be recorded. Questions, answers, hypotheses, probabilities, uncertainty estimates, diagnoses, prescriptions (the latter five noted on a sheet of paper) could easily be traced in their real order and in conformity with the time sequence. The technician was asked to watch over the proceedings.

Three to seven days later, the videotape was commented on by the physi-cian-participants. In the presence of the investigator the physician answered questions about the (face) validity and the reliability of the simulation, the rejection of hypotheses or hypotheses unmentioned, and his estimation of probabilities and uncertainty. He was asked to break down his diagnosis into its characteristic symptoms (signs, tests, etc.). He was then allowed to criticize his procedure and outcome.

The candidate had to solve four patient problems within an hour. Although he was free to choose his time, he was at intervals reminded of the other 'patients' waiting in the waiting room.

Sixty-eight physicians participated in the study: 60 family physicians, 8 general internists. Of the 60 participating family physicians 8 of them solved three patient problems. Six out of these eight family physicians could not complete the simulation because of the urgent calls of real patients: they completed the three patients in an average time of 45 minutes, which is consistent with the average time of the total group. We were conversant with the fact that generally internists take more time per patient in real life. We urged them to do at least three cases, and they all succeeded except one, again for urgent reasons.

The physician's experience of the 'realistic' simulation seems to depend on a number of features such as: surroundings, the presentation of the patient's complaint, the recognition of this complaint as well-known, time constraints, and frequency of questioning and answering. We asked the participants to estimate to what extent the simulation matched the routine practice situation. They denoted their estimation on a five point scale ranging from one – perfectly comparable – to five, uncomparable. The results are shown below.

TABLE 1

Perceived degree of realism of the simulation per case

Scale	Average %
1	62
2	35
3	3
4	–
5	–

The free questioning, the freedom to formulate the question in an accustomed way and in the order the physicians wished and were familiar with, contributed a great deal to this favourable result.

Participants reported that they experienced hardly any difference from 'normal' practising except for the fact that they were often required to explain or specify their questions. The mediator reported that he now had acquired good impression of how patients must feel with these multi-attributed questions of physicians. It was at this point that physicians found simulation to be different from normal duty.

A detailing of these results for the particular patient cases gave almost the same results, ranging from 88–100% preceived realism.

The mediator's task was to answer the physician's questions as accurately and quickly as possible. He had to perform a 'search and find' procedure within an acceptable time schedule. The results are shown in the following table.

Time started after the presentation of the complaint. With regard to the frequency of questioning and answering an average number of three per minute was reported in the literature (Dudley and Blanchard, 1976). In this project we found for family physicians an average of 2.9 questions per minute,

TABLE 2

Response to doctors' questions

	Number	%
Total number of questions asked:	9463	100
Retrievability	9378	99
Questions unanswered	85	1

and for general internists 4.2 questions/minute which underscores the findings of Dudley and Blanchard. A frequency distribution over the cases is showed in the following table.

TABLE 3

Frequency distribution of questions/minute

Questions/minute	Family physicians		General internists	
	Number	Percentage	Number	Percentage
0–1	4	1.7	–	–
1–2	22	9.5	–	–
2–3	93	40.0	2	9.5
3–4	83	35.8	5	24.0
4–5	26	11.3	12	57.1
5–6	1	0.4	1	4.7
6–7	2	0.9	1	4.7
7–8	–	–	–	–
8–9	1	0.4	–	–

As shown in the table the speed of questioning and answering is not influenced by the simulation method. The method can meet speeds of up to 8–9 questions per minute. We did not discern any influence for first or subsequent cases presented to the physician. The order in which cases were presented alternated according to a preconceived scheme.

We asked the participants about their feelings of uncertainty, of being examined, at the beginning and during the simulation. It was hypothesized that mounting feelings of uncertainty would negatively influence the task performance. They noted down this emotion on two five-point scales, one for the start-position, one for the situation during the process, ranging from 1: highly uncertain to 5: very certain, and Ø: no reaction of this kind at all.

The scale was designed from minus 3 to plus 3

−3	−1	0	1	3

highly uncertain   very certain

At the start 23 physician found no unusual reaction. Calculating the responses for the other

Start: Certainty minus Uncertainty = + 2.
During: Certainty minus Uncertainty = + 58.

Most participants said that they felt almost immediately at ease during the session. An important finding was their observation that their uncertainty was not much different from the feelings they experience during normal routine practice.

We asked the participants to score their subjective opinions about the mode of the simulation (with regard to the actual processes). They scored on a 5-points scale indicating: 1: very high resemblance with actual practice work to 5: no relation to practical work; and 0 A: no opinion.

The results were very stimulating. A simulation mode had been created

TABLE 4

Distributions of degrees of perceived realism of simulation mode for 60 family physicians and 8 general internists

Degree of realism (decreasing)	Total	Fam. physcn	Gen. internist
1	27 (40)	25 (42)	2 (25)
2	37 (54)	32 (54)	5 (63)
3	3 (4)	2 (3)	1 (12)
4	–	–	–
5	–	–	–
0	1 (2)	1 (1)	–

(The percentages in parentheses).

which is not only very accurate, easy to produce and highly realistic, but also very much appreciated by the physicians.

Summary

People cannot freely observe without a particular intention or theory in mind. This conception largely determines what we shall see and what we want to see. Most observational research is liable to this bias. To protect oneself against this tendency an explicitly formulated design can help to overcome the bias. A model can serve this purpose. We created two models to cover the inference processes as they might be observed in physicians' problem-solving and decision-making. One model stands for the deductive type of reasoning, the other represents the inductive method. Three subtypes in the inductive method have been distinguished.

The modeling enabled us to formulate the core body and the distinguishing features of these devices. The predictions as based on the (theoretical background of the) models and their criteria could validate these systems towards the real-life situations. Essential to this validation is a standardised input into the system. However, standardisation in medicine is often hard to find. To develop a standardised system which could contain the data from different patient cases was one of the major tasks of the study. The 'paper patient' appeared to be a great success and contributed largely to the realisation of the study.

The hierarchical nesting of the hypotheses as distinctive landmarks within the deductive method required the development of an instrument which could detect the different levels of hypothesis-specification. We delineated five levels of specification ranging from total body definition to a characterisation on the cellular level.

Symptoms, the number of questions, and 'time' functioned as special landmarks which enabled us to detect those specific characteristics that specified the models and the subtypes.

The introduction of verbal communication between the 'patient' and the physician (by means of a physician-mediator) facilitated the investigatory procedure. The procedure took place in the physician's habitual environment, his own office, which also contributed to the success. According to the participants the investigatory procedure approached the real-life situation which not only stimulated the experimenter but the participating physicians as well.

Chapter VI

Results of the study

> Nothing is more difficult to change than the person who thinks he knows exactly what he is doing and why he is doing it.

Introduction

In the preceding chapters we outlined the conceptual framework which leads to the construction of the models, their main characteristics, and the tools to be used to acquire the empirical evidence pertinent to the theory. We distinguished two basic ways of clinical reasoning: the deductive and the inductive type, the latter being subdivided into three methods: pattern recognition, inductive-heuristic, and inductive-algorithmic. We hypothesized that the pattern recognition and the inductive-heuristic methods were mainly used by family physicians, the deductive and the inductive-algorithmic method usually by general internists.

The landmarks within the clinical reasoning methods are formed by:
– hypotheses;
– symptoms;
– questions, and as a corollary;
– time.

The hypotheses can characterize a particular method in three ways: early generation, specification, and redundancy.

Standardized symptoms enabled to nearly perfect comparability as well as tracing the lines of the strategies by means of their attachment to the hypotheses.

The questions could be linked to the data because of the standardization of the structure in which the patient's data were recorded.

As a result of the use of strict definitions the methods could easily be traced and detected. The various predictions within the conceptual framework could be tested using the acquired empirical data. Especially the very personal approach to clinical problems, the personal way of processing the information, the idiosyncratic conceptions of diagnoses and diseases that characterize the inductive reasoning process is a striking characteristic of physicians' behaviour. It exposes physicians, students, teachers, health care managers, politicians, and patients to several difficult problems. It makes it more difficult to introduce decision-aids or knowledge-bases into the day-to-day practice. At least the study elicited a common denominator for clinical reasoning processes. This discovery highlights the need for further study in this area..

The criteria for the strategies

From the description of the models we can now delineate the criteria for the various strategies.

In their psychological model of diagnostic inquiry Elstein and colleagues (1978) used three features to account for medical diagnostic reasoning: information search units, cues, and hypotheses. Cues and hypotheses were used as cross-cutting dimensions in a two-dimensional matrix according to which each simulation was structured. To determine the quality, the effectiveness and the efficiency of the problem-solving process, cues were weighted according to a pre-established arrangement, which was based on expert judgements. Whether an information search unit could be assigned as a cue (a symptom relevant to a diagnostic hypothesis) was arbitrated by experts. Two objections can be made to this procedure. As we discussed before (Chapter I) personal interpretations make unanimity of a disease conception questionable. Interdoctor variation can lead to erroneous cue assignment. Secondly, as symptoms can bear varying meanings and weightings with regard to a particular diagnosis, symptoms can be differently judged especially when they are not standardized. To avoid interpretational bias we searched for objective criteria; criteria which could unambiguously be observed or, preferably, expressed in numerical terms. As mentioned in Chapter V it led to four landmarks in the clinical reasoning process:
- – hypotheses;
- – symptoms
- – number of questions; and
- – time.

With regard to the hypotheses three factors have to be distinguished: their situation within the process (early hypothesis generation), rejection of redundant hypotheses, and the progression down the levels (hierarchical nesting).

Deductive reasoning

In deductive reasoning the landmarks have distinctive characteristics as a result of the requirements of the deductive method (see Chapter II). The generation of a hypothesis must be based on acquired and observed evidence. Therefore, we specified a criterion for a deductive strategy as a certain amount of accumulated evidence (= answers from the patient) ahead of the formulation of the first hypothesis. On empirical grounds we defined this amount as the equivalent of at least 10 answers from the patient. Essential to the deductive method is the formulation of a number of argumentation steps which are represented by a progressive specification of hypotheses. In our investigational situation it meant that the hypotheses as noted down by the participant-physician were formulated within the structure of a one organ system and could be traced in accordance with the preformulated hierarchical levels. Variation of organ systems and reverse hierarchical level indication excluded the deductive method. It also meant that work-ups with less than two hypotheses must be excluded from this method.

The deductive method requires an ultimate proof of the lowest-level hypothesis. It is not compatible with hypotheses that are equally possible. At the end of each work-up the physician was asked if he maintained a hypothesis different from the diagnosis. All cases with more than 1 hypothesis left after the conclusion of the diagnostic process were excluded from the category of deductive strategy.

Recapitulating the criteria for deductive strategy, we have:

(1) DATA COLLECTION. We defined the amount of information collection prior to the first hypothesis as the equivalent of at least 10 answers from the 'patient'.

(2) HYPOTHESIS SPECIFICATION. This criterion is defined as a one-way progression down a number of levels within a particular line of an organ system. This criterion requires a minimum of two hypotheses.

(3) REDUNDANT HYPOTHESES. As a consequence of deductive reasoning the testing of a final (lowest-level) hypothesis can only result in a verification or a falsification. A process which results in a number of equally possible hypotheses is incompatible with deductive reasoning.

Inductive reasoning

It may be recalled that we subdivided the inductive strategy into three types:

(a) pattern recognition;
(b) inductive-heuristic;
(c) inductive-algorithmic.

Pattern recognition

Distinctive to this type is the sudden flash of recognition of a pattern of symptoms on observing only one or two items. It is the 'Aha-Erlebnis' of the recollection of a quite familiar picture one has in mind. Whether this picture is true or false to the facts is not important. It is true to the man or woman who experiences it. We can deduce from this description the following distinctive features:

– the – very – limited amount of data that trigger the 'Aha-Erlebnis';
– the conviction of correctness of the hypothesis.

We define the following criteria for pattern recognition:

(1) NO QUESTIONS may be asked before the generation of the first (and only) hypothesis. We may notice that in our instrument a two-symptoms introduction was automatically introduced. The 'zero' value in the tables refers to active inquiry by the physician;

(2) ONE HYPOTHESIS. As a consequence of the description only one hypothesis is generated. The subject-physician does not consider alternatives.

The next subtype to be distinguished within the inductive way of reasoning is the inductive-heuristic.

Inductive-heuristic

As discussed previously, this type of strategy can be considered as an iterative process on the former theme. In the course of the task performance several patterns as hypotheses jump to mind. These recollections are triggered by some data acquired during the problem-solving. Information and testing cues are completely mixed up and cannot be separated. The hypotheses collected, gradually, form a data base from which in the end the physician picks up one of the hypotheses as a diagnosis. The problem solver regularly visits his 'data base of hypotheses' in order to add a new one or to reconsider the existing ones. The hypotheses do not form a hierarchical structure of levels within a certain organ system, but are randomly generated regardless of levels and organ systems. At the end of the diagnostic process a number of hypotheses is maintained, perhaps in order to fall back on alternative hypotheses in the 'hypotheses base' in case of failing predictive outcomes. From these thoughts we can note down the discriminating criteria for this strategy.
 (1) NO QUESTIONS ahead of the generation of the first hypothesis. The first step in this strategy reflects the pattern recognition mode. In a small minority of cases (six) a limited number of questions was asked in this phase. Because of the following criteria these strategies were enclosed in this subtype.
 (2) HYPOTHESES. As described, a 'hypotheses base', a set of hypotheses, is constructed during the work-up containing a varying number of hypotheses.
 (3) HYPOTHESES LEVELS. Because the hypotheses were generated randomly the levels do not follow a particular line or structure.

Inductive-algorithmic

The last category of our model is the inductive-algorithmic strategy. In many respects it resembles the former strategy. It differs in the method of data collection. While in the former mode the data collection is directed by intuition, the casual answers of the patient, questions arising on the spur of the moment; in this strategy more or less fixed runs of questions are asked; runs of questions covering most of the organ systems regardless of the organ system to which the patient's complaint refers (and to which most of the hypotheses can be attributed). It is a way of superficially screening the patient. It is a kind of habit in which these more or less fixed runs of questions are applied across the various cases. These runs are typically person-bound and can differ in content and order from physician to physician. Distinctive of this type of strategy is the total number of questions, which surpasses greatly the number of questions in the former strategies. On empirical grounds, we found the number of 65 questions as the decisive point in the determination of the criteria, which can be summarized as follows:
 (1) no questions ahead of the first hypothesis;
 (2) more than 1 hypothesis;

(3) hypotheses levels ranging randomly;
(4) more than 65 questions asked.

The research material was searched in a branching fashion. After the search for records in which a deductive strategy might have been applied, we followed the next scheme:

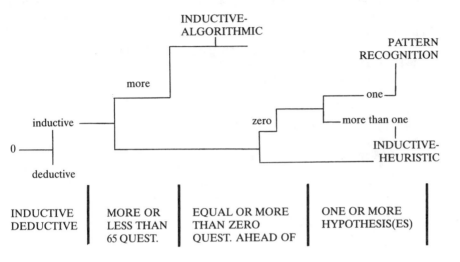

Applying these criteria to the collected data of 253 solved patient cases we found the following results.

(1) Deductive reasoning could not be detected.
(2) All patient cases were solved according to the inductive method.

The distribution of the three sub-methods is as follows:

TABLE 1

Frequency distribution of the inductive strategies

Subtypes	Absolute frequency	Family physicians	General internists	Relative frequency
Pattern recognition	53	52	1	21
Inductive-heuristic	172	168	4	68
Inductive-algorithmic	28	12	16	11

The cyclic and groping method of the inductive-heuristic strategy is the more prevalent method, followed by pattern recognition, the method of the 'clinical vision', the 'flair clinique'. The more time-consuming inductive-algorithmic method is the least prevalent one.

With regard to the various patient cases a predominance of the pattern-recognition subtype can be attributed to the more prevalent kinds of disease like asthmatic-bronchitis (26.7%), atopic eczema (30.3%), and gall-stones (39.4%). Any other preference of a particular disease to a particular method could not be traced.

Any indication of preference by a physician to a particular subtype was sought in vain. More than 60% of the physicians used more than two strategies, changing randomly from one subtype to another. Apparently, not the subtypes but the general concept of inductive reasoning is the common denominator for the clinical method.

As the inductive method represents a personal approach the visualization of this method can only be achieved by picturing this strategy on a case basis. We shall present three cases as solved by three physicians for one disease: iron-deficiency anaemia. The flow of the strategy follows from the time indication in the left-hand column. The meaning of the letter combinations, as explained in Chapter V, shall shortly be recapitulated.

Iron-deficiency anemia

Time/min-utes	Physician A			Physician B			Physician C		
	HPS	HRS	NHRS	HPS	HRS	NHRS	HPS	HRS	NHRS
1	4	–	–	3	–	1	3	1	–
2	–	2	1	1	2	–	2	–	–
3	1	2	2	–	2	2	–	–	1
4	2	2	–	–	–	3	2	1	2
5	1	1	1	–	–	2	2	1	–
6	–	2	–	1	2	2	–	–	5
7	–	3	–	–	1	3	–	–	2
8	–	1	–	1	3	1	3	–	1
9	–	–	3	4	–	–	–	2	2
10	–	–	1	2	–	3	–	2	1
11				–	–	5	–	–	6
12				–	–	1	–	4	1
13				1	–	1	–	3	2
14				2	–	–	–	5	–
15				1	–	–	–	–	1

16	–	1	–	–	–	1
17	–		3			
18	–	4	1			
19	–	1	4			
20	–	2	2			
21	–	1	3			

HPS   = Hypotheses Pre-related Symptom(s), which is (are) the symptom(s) preceding to the generation of a hypothesis.

HRS   = Hypothesis Related Symptom(s), which is (are) a kind of 'testing' of symptoms following a formulated hypothesis.

NHRS = Non-Hypothesis Related Symptom(s); as the word suggests, it denotes (a) symptoms not related to any hypothesis.

The various signs mean:

▭   = hypothesis;

⊞   = diagnostic hypothesis; a hypothesis within the trail of hypotheses, which in the end is picked as the diagnosis;

⊟@   = diagnosis.

The numbers in the columns refer to the number of symptoms (per time-unit)

These examples show a number of characteristics of the inductive reasoning processes.

- As can be predicted by the model of inductive reasoning the first hypothesis is generated immediately after the initial presentation of the complaints (2 clinical items) as is shown by the example of doctor C.
- Even in the case of more elaborate questioning the first hypothesis is formulated after only a few more clinical data as is demonstrated by physicians A and B.
- Information acquisition towards the formulation of a hypothesis as represented by HPS and clinical data which can serve as the test of such a formulated hypothese, represneted by HRS, are completely mixed during the work-up. This is in conformity with the theory of inductive reasoning (see Medawar, 1969).
- The pace of questioning varies greatly during the work-up of the case. The numbers of questions vary from 1 per minute to 5 or 6. From our material we found a variable pacing of questioning which reflected the physician's habitual working pattern.
- A final choice (diagnosis) may be made among the hypotheses collected during the process as is demonstrated by the processes of physicians B and C (the first respectively the fourth hypothesis is chosen as the diagnosis). It has the appearance of a haphazard choice but we conjecture a weighing of the acquired hypotheses according to personal standards and beliefs (experience).
- The personal belief in the final statement is demonstrated by the non-testing of the diagnosis (physician A with none and physician C with one

Non-hypothesis-related symptom). We have to realize that in the case of physician B the final choice at the end of the work-up was not followed by any testing. Indeed, in all 253 work-ups of the patient cases any testing of a diagnosis will be sought in vain.

- In the cases of physicians B and C the process seems to goon and on, data acquisition – hypothesis generation – data acquisition-hypothesis generation, etc. Apparently, time sets constraints to this process.[1]

Relevancy and redundancy in information processing

In the literature (Lindley, 1975; Knill-Jones, 1975; Gill *et al.*, 1973; Pipberger *et al.*, 1968) on decision-making the physician's inefficiency of information processing is exemplified by the redundancy of the amount of information needed to arrive at a diagnosis. This judgement, however, can only be made with hindsight. Nobody, unless one is aware of the definite diagnosis, can tell us beforehand which datum can contribute to a particular diagnosis and which not. The collection of data typically reflects the trial-and-error method of the physician, formulating a number of possible solutions. As we could connect the symptoms to the pertinent hypothesis we were able to judge the relevancy as well as the redundancy of the symptoms with regard to a particular hypothesis. The HPS and HRS typically represent the relevant symptoms, the NHRS the 'redundant' symptoms.

TABLE 2

Frequency distribution of relevant and redundant symptoms (mean values)

Hypothesis pre-related symptoms		Hypothesis related symptoms		Total related symptoms	Redundant symptoms	
Number	%	Number	%	%	Number	%
16.4	19	47.12	53	72	24.9	28

From these figures it may be clear that redundancy is not a prominent feature of the physician's reasoning process. Moreover, it would be less than reassuring if physicians did not make efforts to explore the patient's 'data base' in different directions in order to find appropriate cues. An average percentage of 28% seems very reasonable to meet the complex task of finding relevant cues in an unknown 'data base'.

By comparison we can assume a higher 'redundancy' in the algorithmic mode. To enable this comparison we standardized the numbers of symptoms for the specific strategies. The results are shown in the following table.

---

[1] (These conclusions are, as a matter of fact, based on the complete material of the study).

The relevancy of symptoms pertinent to the problem-solving process can be expressed by the so-called *relevancy factor*. This factor can be expressed as

TABLE 3

Frequency distribution of related and redundant symptoms for two strategies

Strategy	Standard number of symptoms	Mean related	Mean redundant
Heuristic	100	74.7	25.3
Algorithmic	100	67.6	32.4

The outcomes follow our prediction of higher redundancy for the algorithmic mode.

$$\frac{HPS + HRS}{HPS + HRS + NHRS} \times 100.$$

As it represents the relationship between hypotheses and symptoms, it may provide some indication of the progression from formulating to testing the hypotheses in the diagnostic process. It is generally assumed that experienced people use less data to generate and test a hypothesis/diagnosis than a novice, while novices have a more indeterminate search for symptoms. It means that the relevancy factor scores higher for experienced physicians than for novices or students. The average relevancy factor was calculated at 73.72. The calculation for physicians with less than 5 years experience in clinical practice came to 69.78; for experienced physicians, those with more than 20 years practice, the figure was 76.21. These figures fall within the range of chance and so do not permit one to draw any conclusions. It may suggest that the factor is too crude to measure these assumed differences; or the differences as they are insinuated follow more from 'common sense' reasoning than from firm evidence; or experience is acquired much faster than we suppose. It would be very in-

TABLE 4

Relevancy factors for the different patient cases

Patient case	Relevancy factor
(1) Myocardial infarction	79.22
(2) Sciatica	73.68
(3) Atopic eczema	76.28
(4) Extra-uterine pregnancy	79.83
(5) Gall-stones	83.21
(6) Hyperthyroidism	61.29
(7) Asthmatic bronchitis	85.29
(8) Iron-deficiency anaemia	69.37

The relevancy factor shows little variation across the cases. Apparently, this factor cannot be related to the difficulty of the problem.

teresting to relate this factor to the problem-solving exercises of medical students as compared to 'experienced' physicians.

When the relevancy factor was related to the various patient cases little variation was found to exist.

Apparently, this relevancy factor cannot be related to the nature of the problem. On the other hand, it exhibits a consistent distribution within the medical problem-solving task.

On hypotheses

Hypotheses are considered to be the cornerstones in the reasoning processes. They are usually not the logical stepping stones towards diagnosis as conjectured; they seem to represent the analogies to remembered cases, the mental patterns as they are sensed from one or two presented symptoms. They allow the physician to narrow the size of the problem space; they also help him to overcome the inherent limitations in the thinking process (which are discussed in Chapter III).

In the 253 problem-solving tasks used in this study 745 hypotheses were generated, including the diagnoses. 90% of the first hypotheses were formulated immediately after the symptoms were presented (no questions from the physician). According to the literature problem-solving processes should be case dependent, i.e., more complicated and more time-consuming with increasing difficulty. We defined the odd numbered cases as the easier ones, and, conversely, the others as the difficult ones because of their low appearance in the population. With regard to the number of hypotheses we could not detect any 'problem-orientation' for high or low prevalence cases. On average the numbers ranged between 3.0 and 4.3 hypotheses per case randomly distributed over high and low prevalent cases.

In regard to the hierarchical nesting of hypotheses in a deductive inference process we designed a device for recognizing these levels according to progressive specification of body-parts and systems. For convenient reasons we shall recapitulate these levels:

Level I   : All matters affecting the total human body;
Level II   : Multiorganic Formulation: diseases and illnesses concerning body systems and/or body parts;
Level III : Organ systems. The nomenclature following the usual medical classification;
Level IV   : Organ. Diseases and illnesses of specific organs;
Level V   : 'Cellular Level': the main diagnostic entity, the most specified biopathological state.

Because we could not detect any deductive strategy, a pattern of hierarchical nesting was sought in vain. The inductive method predicts the opposite of hierarchical nesting: a wide variability in the degree of specification of hypotheses within a diagnostic process.[2] The degrees of specification of the hypotheses are shown in the following table.

The 745 hypotheses were distributed over the levels as follows.

---

[2] We have to realize that any hierarchical nesting can only be deduced from singular cases.

TABLE 5

Frequency distribution of hypotheses over the levels

Level	No. of hypotheses	Percentage
I	30	4
II	100	13
III	110	15
IV	229	31
V	276	37
Total	745	100

The predicted variability of hypotheses-specification is clearly demonstrated in this table. It underlines the inductive character of the problem-solving method.

The distribution mirrors satisfactorily the expected numbers of hypotheses within the predefined levels. It has to be realized that the more precise the specification of the various body- and tissue compartments the more patho-(physio)logical entities can be defined. We had expected some linearity of the percentages through the levels. Apparently, this is not the case, which can be due either to the definition of the levels or to the less specified nomenclature of the physicians. If the former is the case we may expect a rise in numbers for the high(er) level hypotheses, the ones that serve as diagnoses. We therefore manipulated the material in such a way that diagnoses could be temporarily recognized as 'last hypotheses' for reasons of comparability. The following table shows the results.

TABLE 6

Distribution of the levels for the first and last hypotheses

	First hypotheses					Last hypotheses				
	I	II	III	IV	V	I	II	III	IV	V
No.	15	44	35	85	74	2	18	27	88	118
%	6	17	14	34	29	1	7	11	34	45

There are some tendencies towards higher-level hypotheses. These shifts are within chance distribution.

For the ultimate diagnoses the following percentages were found for the various levels.

Although some tendency towards higher-level hypotheses can be noticed, these shifts are small and do not exceed chance variability. We suppose that the lack of specified diagnostic nomenclature is the main cause of the variability. This phenomenon can be illustrated by listing the nomenclature of the diagnoses for the eight different cases. It was to be expected that some variation of nomenclature would exist due, for example to diagnostic error.

TABLE 7

Distribution of the levels for the diagnoses of the eight cases

	Level				
	I	II	III	IV	V
No.	2	18	27	100	106
%	0.8	7	11	40	42

However, we found more than 75 different diagnostic names for eight different patient cases. This was far more than we had anticipated. The relatively high amount of low-level diagnostic names was surprising. The following table gives the overall results.

TABLE 8

Differences of diagnostic nomenclature

	Level				
	I	II	III	IV	V
No.	2	18	27	100	106
Diff. nom.	2	14	18	28	15
%	100	78	67	28	14

The lack of standard medical nomenclature is demonstrated in this table. On level II 14 different names for 18 diagnoses and 18 different names for 27 diagnoses on level III are ominous signs for uniformity and generalization of medical knowledge. In the more specified sectors the numbers are less dramatic.

We found 250 different names among the 745 hypotheses. The verbally creative possibilities of the physician seem to be inexhaustible. Columns and columns were filled with fancy names. It gives one an uneasy feeling in regard to the consistency and the use of an unanimous language in medicine.

This variation in nomenclature was a reason to search for another kind of variability: the variation of the hypotheses over the different human organ systems. As reported in Chapter V we distinguished nine various organ systems (and another two because they were erroneously mentioned by the participant).[3] For every patient case we found on average that the hypotheses varied over five different organ systems (minimally 4, maximally 8). Possible problem-orientation might exist because the so-called low-prevalent cases varied on average over seven different systems as compared to four for the high-prevalent diseases.

These figures may erroneously give the impression that physicians are 'wild guessers'. However, this impression is not quite justified. The physician often

[3] (10) psychosocial system; and (11) undetermined somatic disease.

has to deal with symptoms overlapping more than one organ system. For instance, the symptom dyspnea (breathlessness) can refer to both the cardiac and respiratory dysfunction. Taking into consideration the appropriate organ system and its adjacent one the relevancy of the hypotheses to the presented case can be shown in table 9.

TABLE 9

Relevancy of hypotheses per patient case as proportional to the total number of hypotheses per case

Patient	1	2	3	4	5	6	7	8
Hypoth. pert.	68	44	82	74	90	48	90	35
Hypoth. adj.	18	40	15	21	7	9	4	4
Total	86	84	97	95	97	57	94	39

Generally speaking, doctors continue to focus on the organ system and its adjacent one as being the right ones. Variability must be largely attributed to the meanings of the various symptoms.

Cases 6 and 8 seem to represent the exception. Perhaps physicians need some pretext, thus far hidden from our observations, to become 'wild guessers'.

From our inquiry we learned that problem-orientation was less related to the specific disease than to the presented symptoms. When symptoms such as 'tiredness', 'feeling ill', etc., were mentioned early in the work-up, some physicians reacted adversely, as if they did not know what to do with this kind of information. As problem-orientation was consistently found in problem-solving procedures (see, e.g., Newell and Simon, 1972), it seems quite possible that problem-orientation is more intimately related to the presenting of symptoms than to (the prevalence of the) disease.

A final remark about hypotheses concerns the rejection of hypotheses. As we have mentioned, rejection of hypotheses is not an innate trait of the inductive strategy, as opposed to the deductive strategy. We found for the relevant strategies (pattern-recognition was excluded because of its one-hypothesis feature) a rejection rate on the average of 0.8. Less than 1 hypothesis was rejected, so that we can calculate a hypothesis-redundancy of (on average) 77% hypotheses per case. We need to emphasize that 'rejection' has different meanings for the deductive and the inductive method. In the deductive strategy the rejection is a result of experimental testing of the evidence at hand in order to falsify the hypothesis; the hypothesis becomes untenable. In the inductive process the hypothesis loses its relevancy, not as a result of negative test results but as a loss of belief, conviction, on the part of the physician. Its probability estimate falls below a – personally defined – threshold. This threshold can vary from physician to physician, from case to case, from day to day.

On symptoms and diagnoses

If a hypothesis is conceived as a cluster of symptoms[4] it is interesting to know whether these clusters are consistent across the various physicians who generated the same hypothesis. Traditionally, the configuration of symptoms has defined a particular disease. By means of its specific symptom-pattern one disease can be distinguished from another. When one knows and remembers the specific pattern the accurate diagnosis can be made. However, as the concept of a disease is rather vague and can vary among physicians, so many of the patterns of symptoms can similarly differ. Besides, symptom-patterns are by no means fixed but can differ within a certain range from patient to patient, from situation to situation, from time to time, as every doctor is well aware. As physicians accustomed to use abstract names for our diagnostic nomenclature, much of the inconsistency of the symptom-configurations is hidden from observation.

We used two ways to gain insight into the configurational elements of diagnostic entities:

(1)   aggregations of symptoms which could be connected to the diagnosis (respectively the diagnostic hypothesis) during the work-up of the case (symptom clustering);

(2)   after the doctor had arrived at a diagnosis we asked him to specify this disease-entity in the way he had memorized it from medical school, textbooks, etc., and employed it as such (decomposition procedure).

We shall deal with these two approaches successively.

Symptom clustering

We collected all homonymous diagnoses as made by the participating physicians. Each doctor solved approximately 4 patient cases, which were randomly allocated to the physicians. It meant that each patient-case was presented approximately 32 times.[5]

Only different symptoms were included, which meant that when homonymous symptoms were asked about more than once by one physician they were only included as that particular symptom. So we got for one disease which was diagnosed by 'p' physicians 'q' number of symptoms. These elements were arranged into a matrix with the codes for the separate symptoms in columns and the codes for the physicians in rows. Within this matrix we performed a re-arrangement programme which brought the most prevalent symptoms (asked at least five times by the group of physicians) to the left hand upper corner of the matrix, and in succession less prevalent symptoms in the right hand lower-corner. Consequently, the right hand lower corner remained almost empty. This re-arrangement created a kind of 'most-prevalent' space within the matrix, as is shown in the following scheme.

---

[4] 'Symptoms' understood as in the definition in Chapter V.

[5] Some variation was due to unfinished sessions.

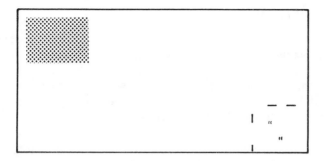

We shall present the statistics of four examples.

Example 1. Myocardial infarction
23 subjects asked 283 symptoms of which 58 were distinct. We found for the 'most-prevalent' symptoms a number 11, asked by 12 subjects. It meant that the 'most-prevalent symptoms-space' could be calculated as being 9.9% of the total area of symptoms. However, the coverage within this 'space' was not complete. Only 69 (52%) out of the possible 132 symptoms were included in this space.

Example 2. Asthmatic bronchitis
18 subjects asked 229 symptoms of which 56 were distinct. The number of 'most-prevalent' symptoms was 14, asked by 15 subjects. The 'most-prevalent-symptom-space' was 20%. The coverage within the space was 74 (35%) out of the possible 210 symptoms.

Example 3. Hyperthyroidism
27 subjects asked 543 symptoms of which 115 symptoms were distinct. The number of 'most-prevalent' symptoms was 28, asked by 23 physicians. The 'most-prevalent-symptom-space' was 20%. The coverage within the space was 187 (29%) out of the possible symptoms.

Example 4. Iron-deficiency anemia
25 subjects asked 407 symptoms of which 93 symptoms were distinct. The number of the 'most-prevalent' symptoms was 22, asked by 22 physicians. The 'most-prevalent-symptom-space' was 20%. The coverage within the space was 131 (27%) out of the 484 possible symptoms.

These examples were chosen because they represent different types of diseases and allowed these calculations. In the majority of cases the symptoms varied so much that no real matrices or 'spaces' could be found or created.

Within this material we have calculated that the chance of a particular symptom pertinent to a disease being also incorporated into the work-up of a colleague is less than 1%.

Decomposition procedure

After they had made a diagnosis we asked the participating physicians to delineate the composing elements of the diagnosis they had just made in order to denote the picture of the symptom configuration which they had in mind. They all pictured the particular disease as they saw it in terms of a number of symptoms. Obviously, one can distinguish two types of consistency regarding these elements: external and internal consistency.

External consistency indicates the agreement on symptoms among physicians concerning the same disease. For instance, when 10 physicians make the diagnosis Myocardial Infarction, the question is on how many symptoms do they agree in making that particular diagnosis.

Internal consistency refers to the matching – by the physicians – of the given picture of the disease and the actual acquired symptoms during the work-up.

External consistency factor
First we shall deal with external consistency. For example, with a particular diagnosis a large number of symptoms concerning this diagnosis have been named. Some of these symptoms are mentioned by all physicians who have diagnosed this disease (= 100% external consistency). Other symptoms are only mentioned by half of these physicians (= 50% external consistency) or a quarter (= 25%) and so on. When a number of symptoms is mentioned for a particular disease each of the symptoms has a corresponding percentage related to the number of physicians who have asked about the symptom. The sum of these percentages divided by the total number of different symptoms constitute the *mean external consistency factor*.
   The *mean external consistency factor* can be defined as:

> the average with which any symptom within a cluster of symptoms, corresponding to a particular disease, is mentioned within a group of physicians who asked about these symptoms.

With the exception of the atopic eczema case (where hardly any common denominator could be found), all patient cases exhibit similar patterns. We shall, therefore, present only three examples: one for sciatica, one for chole-lithiasis (gall-stones), and one for extra-uterine pregnancy.
   In the tables the symptoms are denoted by a letter code. For the leading symptoms we shall present a decoding. The numbers refer to the times this particular symptom is mentioned within the group of physicians who diagnosed the same disease. The percentages in the third row indicate the external consistency for that particular symptom.

Example 1. Sciatica
The number of physicians who arrived at this diagnosis was 17. The number of depicted symptoms totals 56 of which 24 were distinct. Eight symptoms were

more or less shared within the group of physicians. One symptom was shared by all participants leading to an external consistency of 100%; other symptoms achieved lower ratings. The results are listed in the following table.

TABLE 10(a)

External consistency

Decomposition of the diagnoses into their symptoms; consensus of opinion about these symptoms among the physicians

Sciatica

Number of physicians with the same diagnosis: 17
Total number of symptoms: 56

Symptoms	A	B	C	D	E	F	G	H	I	
Number	17	8	4	3	2	2	2	2	1	(16×)
%	100	47	24	18	12	12	12	12	–	

Mean external consistency factor: 9.9.

For only three symptoms could a more consistent picture within the group of participating physicians be found. The other symptoms hardly rose beyond the level of coincidental agreement.
Leading symptoms: A: pain; B: achilles tendon reflex; C: lower extremity sensory loss.

Example 2. Gall-stones
The number of physicians who arrived at the same diagnosis was 21. The total number of symptoms mentioned was 87 of which 26 were distinct.

TABLE 10(b)

Cholelithiasis (gall-stones)

Number of physicians with the same diagnosis: 21.
Total number of symptoms: 87.

Symptoms	A	B	C	D	E	F	G	H	I	J	K	L	
Number	21	13	9	8	5	4	4	2	2	2	2	1	(15×)
%	100	62	43	38	24	19	19	9	9	9	9	–	

Mean external consistency factor: 13.1.

For only five symptoms was some consistency of the symptom configuration of the diagnosis found. We consider an external consistency of less than 20% as mere chance.
Leading symptoms: A: pain; B: food intolerance; C: discoloration of stools.

Example 3. Extra-uterine pregnancy
Twenty-four physicians arrived at this diagnosis and chose a total of 100 symptoms of which 32 were distinct.

TABLE 10(c)

Extra-uterine pregnancy

Number of physicians with the same diagnosis: 24.
Total number of symptoms: 100.

Symptoms	A	B	C	D	E	F	G	H	J	K	L	M	
Number	22	15	11	8	6	5	4	2	2	2	2	1	(21×)
%	92	63	46	33	25	21	17	8	8	8	8	–	

Mean external consistency factor: 10.0.

Leading symptoms: A: pain; B: menstrual cycle alteration; C: perspiration.

From our theory of inductive reasoning we conjectured that every physician carries his own idea, his own stereotype of a disease. To test this theory we asked the physician-participants to decompose their stereotype into the constituent parts of the disease they had just diagnosed, the specific symptom-pattern they had in mind. The mean external consistency factor illustrates the consensus of opinion within a group of doctors with regard to their description of the symptom-patterns of a particular disease. This factor has been calculated at 10% which means that within a group of physicians agreement on the specific components of a symptom-pattern does not exceed one symptom for every 10 mentioned. In our material we found that the physicians agreed on only one symptom in their joint disease-descriptions. Obviously, a name of a disease can be conceived only as a very individualistic concept which can cover a wide variety of meanings.

This striking phenomenon can be considered as a serious obstacle to the identification and classification of diseases. It means that there are grave limitations to the construction of data-bases when they are based on unscreened input of physicians' judgements.

The internal consistency factor compares the physician's stereotype (the decomposition of the diagnosis into symptoms and signs) with his actual data acquisition from the patient scenario. Following our theory of induction we concluded that we could not guarantee any disease description as accurate. This thought implied that every doctor has his own right to his idiosyncratic disease description, his own stereotype. Any comparison between the physician's process and the diagnosis, therefore, must be based on a comparison of individual standards. Secondly, we guessed that the doctor's description of the disease does not necessarily imply that he actually will collect all the data incorporated in his disease description.

The average disease description contained 4.5 symptoms. Comparing the disease description with the actual work-up of the case revealed a discrepancy between the description and the collected clinical data. The internal consistency factor describes this discrepancy. It answers the question: 'how consistent is the doctor with his own memorized picture?' The next table gives some results for a number of diseases.

TABLE 11

Internal consistency
or
'How consistent is the physician's picture?'

Diagnosis	No. of depicted symptoms (mean values)	No. of symptoms (mean values)	Internal consistency %
Myocard. inf.	4.7	2.8	60
Sciatica	3.3	1.9	58
Cholelithiasis	4.1	2.7	66
Hyperthyroid.	5.7	3.9	68
Asthm. bronch.	5.2	3.0	58
Extra-ut. preg.	4.2	3.1	74
Iron-def. anaem.	4.6	3.2	70

The disease description contained on average 4.5 symptoms. In the actual work-up the physician collected, on average, 2.9 of the symptoms mentioned in the memorized picture. It means that the internal consistency factor for these diseases can be calculated as 64% (mean value).

The physician's picture of the diagnosis consists on average of 4–5 symptoms. In his work-up he gathers 2–3 of these symptoms. Apparently, two-thirds of the (diagnostic cluster of) symptoms is necessary to make the doctor decide upon a particular diagnosis. The internal consistency factor delineates the discrepancy.

Presumably, this, factor is empirically founded, and based on the – often extreme – variability known to the physicians to exist in disease presentation. Maybe it is this variation of disease presentation together with the capriciousness of nature which leads physicians to the use of inductive strategies and a personal-based medical knowledge.

On questions, answers, and time

Physicians work mostly under pressure of time. 'The essence of the physician's art actually is to make decisions, a tremendous number every day, often on the basis of insufficient evidence, under pressure of time (. . .) and to make them with – at least outwardly – the appearance of a calm, dedicated and warmly human personality' (Biörck, 1977). Some kind of tension exists between the acquisition of a particular amount of information and the available time. According to Biörck the pressure of time leads the doctor to less optimal information acquisition. In any event, a simulation procedure which does not take into account customary time constraints does not reflect actual clinical problem-solving. However, the experimenter has to be aware of certain circumstances inherent in the investigational mode. For instance, the notation of several details (hypotheses, estimates, etc.), the required specification of the question, and last but not least the fact of being observed, add some delay to the process. We estimated the average time for a routine patient-physician contact at approximately 10 minutes for the family physician. Adding another

5 minutes for making notes, explanation and different situation seemed reasonable. On this basis we presented four patient cases to be solved in an hour. Although general internists generally claim half an hour for each patient, we tried to persuade them to perform at high speed, which usually meant three patients within the hour.

As family physicians practise in primary health care they usually face patient populations which are different from those of general internists, who operate customarily in the second line when the first screening of the patient has already been performed. The task-environment of the family physician obviously differs from that of the general internist. It seems reasonable that the family physician, being under more pressure of time, adopted a slightly different problem-solving behaviour. The family physician takes less time for the patient and asks fewer questions. This behaviour can be quite appropriate to the situation in which he practises. A global selection of patients can be life-saving for those individuals who need immediate medical attention, while other problems can be postponed to more suitable times. General internists, on the other hand, practise (as is the case in the Netherlands) amongst a patient population that primarily referred by a family physician. The family physician is in this situation the gate-keeper to the more specialised parts of the clinical health care system. The general internist is consulted after screening and diagnosing of the patient. His approach to problems can be viewed in this context.

As was stated by the physicians and also observed in the study, the participants did not in fact change their practising habits. The figures on questions and time, therefore, almost certainly reflect the actual situation in practice (that is, for first consultation contacts). As might have been clear from the description of the 'paper patient' the clinical data obtained from physical examination and laboratory, X-ray reports, etc., had to be specifically asked for by the physician. The specific datum was then communicated. So, 'questions' include the whole range of clinical data from patients.

We found the following relationships between questioning and time.

TABLE 12

Average number of questions – average times per patient case

	Questions	Time
Fam. physicians	34 ± 12	11.3 ± 4
Gen. internists	81 ± 21	19.3 ± 6

The time is in minutes.

Considerable variation was found. This can be accounted for by at least two components: the range of patient cases used and the different working-patterns of the physicians. Nevertheless, these figures give some indication.

Among the various subtypes of inductive reasoning, pattern-recognition had the lowest values. The average number of questions per case for pattern-recognition was 22 and the average time per case was 7 minutes. These figures were largest for the algorithmic mode: 83 questions/case and 22 minutes/case.

The variation across the patient cases can be attributed to the varying difficulty of the cases (problem-orientation). It has been hypothesized that similar ranges and mean lengths of patient interview suggest similar distributions of case difficulty and complexity (Morrel, 1972). It means a relationship between case-complexity and length of work-up, in which the length of the work-up must be perceived as a question/time relationship. Standardizing the problem case, on the one hand, to the least number of questions and, on the other, to the shortest length of time used in solving the problem, we could construct correction factors for each of the eight patient cases.

The relationship between questions and time can now be calculated crosswise. When the mean number of questions is corrected for the time factor and the mean time (the time used for patient interviewing) is corrected for the number of questions, we may expect an ironing out of the differences between the patient cases in the event of a complete relationship. The result of this operation is shown in Table 13.

TABLE 13

Interrelationship questions – time per patient case

Patient	Questions corrected	Time corrected
1	26.44	7.43
2	23.07	8.52
3	22.63	8.67
4	19.40	10.11
5	23.07	8.50
6	23.69	8.30
7	29.27	6.71
8	21.23	9.24

The differences make clear that the relationship is much more complex than might have been expected. The various deviations remain unexplained. The number on which these calculations are based does not allow for exact conclusions on the subject; it suggests further investigation.

Patient cases 2, 4, 6, and 8 were assumed to be the more difficult cases (middle to low ranking prevalence) when compared to the odd numbered cases. The suggestion of Morrell does not follow from these figures. We can think of several explanations: (i) difficulty and complexity of cases is unrelated to lengths of work-ups: (ii) the relationship is far more complicated than is assumed; (iii) our perception of difficulty and complexity is not connected with prevalence or incidence statistics.

With regard to question/time relationships another important point draws our attention. De Dombal noted: 'The doctor has to ask the right questions, he also has to ask the questions right' (1978). Whether 'our' doctors asked their questions correctly was beyond the scope of the investigation; they all faced an intelligent patient responding to all questions, even the unclear ones, or, in case of doubt, rephrasing the doctor's question to a clear one. Such an ideal situation is certainly not always met with in daily practice. But the first part of de Dombal's remark pertains to the effectiveness of the physician's questioning. Apart from the time constraints this effectiveness includes two components:

– the relation of the questions to the appropriate hypothesis;
– how many times a positive symptom is elicited by a question.

(As mentioned in Chapter I, page 12: the power of positive response is more than 100 times greater than a negative one for a single attribute (Blois, 1983)).

A 'positive symptom' is defined as:

> 'a characteristic of the patient which deviates from normal functioning or form as perceived by patient or physician.'

When the symptom asked for is present in the patient's 'data-base' it is coded as positive; when not present it is coded as negative. With the help of this coding, we could assess the physician's questioning for this type of effectiveness. The following table shows the overall results.

TABLE 14

Proportional number of 'positive symptoms' per total number of questions

	Family physicians	General internists
No. of Pos. Symptoms	4242	596
No. of Questions	7796	1667
Percentage	54.4%	35.8%

The acquisition of 'positive' symptoms appears more effective with family physicians than with general internists.

Family physicians, using predominantly the heuristic version of the inductive method, relate their interviewing questions to the answer of the patient. They reach a higher score for eliciting 'positive symptoms' within a certain time frame when compared with the general internists, who chiefly

TABLE 15

Proportional number of 'positive symptoms' per strategy

Strategy	Pos. sympt. p. physician	No. of physicians	Proportional to total no. of questions	Total no. of questions
Patt. recogn.	15.2	53	58%	1386
Induct.-heur.	18.7	172	55.9%	5765
Induct.-algorith.	28.9	28	35%	2312

The proportional numbers for the acquisition of 'positive symptoms' are favourable for the pattern recognition and the heuristic methods.

employ the inductive-algorithmic strategy. In this latter version the interviewer is less dependent on patients' answers, and is, therefore, less likely to score 'positive symptoms' within the same time frame.

Effectiveness as the ratio of 'positive symptoms' divided by the total number of questions, i.e., the RATIO effectiveness, is highest in the pattern-recognition strategy and lowest in the inductive-algorithmic. But the number of elicited 'positive symptoms', the CONTENT effectiveness, is highest in the inductive-algorithmic strategy and lowest in the pattern-recognition method. It seems that RATIO effectiveness and CONTENT effectiveness operate in opposite directions. It looks as if a physician has to make a choice: a high speed of questioning in order to collect randomly a sufficient number of 'positive symptoms', or the careful selection of questions in the search for cues at a (much) lower speed. In my opinion, physicians are hardly ever aware of this choice. In fact, they act according to their natural behaviour and on the spur of the moment.

An additional investigation of genuine physician-patient contacts revealed that general internists indeed use a more or less fixed series of questions regardless of the problem at hand. They are in a way doing a kind of general screening of the patient apart from paying specific attention to the patient's complaints. The 'fixed series' carry a very personal mark and cannot be viewed as general clinical algorithms. Family physicians act in a quite different way. Their questions are directly connected to the patient's answer. In this way none of these interviews or physical examinations indicates any generality whatsoever, for all are quite unique. In this respect our attention is drawn to a particular observation. It occurred that in response to a vague answer of the patient the following question of the physician was of a broad, general character. This led to some indistinct answer of the patient which in its turn induced a fuzzy question from the doctor and so on, until the interviews ceased for lack of conversation.

However, we have to realize that another feature of the process can be involved. It might be possible that the first steps in the process are more difficult than the later ones. In that case, the physician with the least number of questions runs the risk of eliciting 'positive symptoms' than the persistant physician, who asks questions at great length. We calculated the ratio effectiveness for each block of 10 questions in the order of their questioning.

It may be possible that one of the factors that influences the termination of the physician patient encounter can be attributed to the decreasing output of 'cues'. With regard to the time restrictions, to which every physician is subjected a 'cost-benefit analysis' of the process could, probably unconsciously, play a part.

The content effectiveness is remarkably harmonious across the patient cases.

As is the case in most instances also the content effectiveness seems rather unaffected by the problem complexity.

In general, these results suggest that problem difficulty does not influence the acquisition of 'positive symptoms'. Whether the number of 'positive symp-

TABLE 16

The course of the ratio-effectiveness during the problem-solving

Block of 10 questions	Total number of questions	No. of positive symptoms	Ratio effectiveness %
1–10	4916	3060	62.2
11–20	2265	1115	49.2
21–30	1098	475	43.2
31–40	444	162	36.5
41–50	228	79	34.6
51–60[a]	135	47	34.8

[a] beyond 60 questions calculations become unreliable.

The decreasing numbers of questions is overtaken by the rate of decrease of the 'positive symptoms'. In fact, ratio effectiveness gradually diminishes during the work-up.

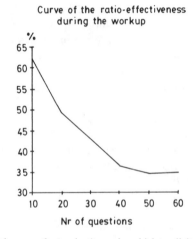

Curve of the ratio-effectiveness during the workup

Evidently, the first questions are the 'easiest' ones by which to elicit positive symptoms. Gradually, the effectiveness levels down to a range between 30 and 35%. This is not a self-evident perspective because the physician cannot foresee the distribution of positive symptoms within a patient 'data-base'.

toms' affects the strategy and the diagnostic outcome is a question for future research.

Each patient scenario had a more or less standardized number of 'positive symptoms' and symptom-aspects (see Chapter V). We did not differentiate between symptom-aspects. Clusters of symptom-aspects were too accidentally achieved, and, therefore, could not contribute to more general features of the process.

When a symptom was asked more than once, partly because of the different aspects, partly because the physician obviously had forgotten the answer, we noted as positive the times the physician asked this special item.

It is the physician's task to elicit effectively the 'positive symptoms and symptom-aspects' from the 'data base', which can be a real-life patient as well

TABLE 17

Content-effectiveness per physician per patient case

Patient case	Number of positive symptoms	Content effectiveness per physician (mean values)
1	547	17.7
2	598	19.3
3	565	17.1
4	804	24.4
5	619	18.7
6	635	19.8
7	517	17.2
8	553	18.4

The content effectiveness shows rather harmonious values across the patient cases.

as a simulated one. The effectiveness of this eliciting leads to the retrieval rate of the questioning process.

TABLE 18

Retrieval rate for 'positive symptoms' from a patient data base

Patient case	Patient data base		Retrieval rate for	
	Symptoms	Symptom-aspects	Symptoms	Symptom-aspects
1	47	278	37.7%	6.5%
2	49	281	39.4%	6.9%
3	54	306	31.7%	5.6%
4	53	316	46.0%	7.7%
5	46	274	40.7%	6.8%
6	48	291	41.3%	6.8%
7	51	293	33.7%	5.9%
8	49	299	37.6%	6.2%

Column 2 displays the standardized numbers of symptoms as they are incorporated into each patient scenario. Column 3 displays the symptom-aspects. The retrieval rate indicates that a relatively large portion of the symptoms in the data base is visited, but in a superficial way, as we can see from the last column.

The retrieval rate relates the acquisition of positive symptoms to the standardized patient scenario. It establishes the thoroughness of searching through this symptom/symptom-aspects data base. Like the content effectiveness it shows a rather harmonious picture across the cases.

The eliciting of symptom-aspects is, according to these results, not a major characteristic of the search procedure. Evidently, a large number of symptoms is visited during the questioning and physical examination (or laboratory data) but only very few symptoms are more deeply interrogated. It gives the impression of skimming-off the territory.

Recapitulating the variables for the positive symptom elicitation we can distinguish three types.

RATIO EFFECTIVENESS relates the acquired number of 'positive symptoms' per case to the total number of questions asked within this case work-up.

CONTENT EFFECTIVENESS relates the number of 'positive symptoms' to the physician who collected them. The figures are given as mean values for a group of physicians solving the same problem. In this respect this variable allows comparison of effectiveness of cue acquisition between physicians.

RETRIEVAL RATE relates the collected number of 'positive symptoms' per case to the standardized patient data base. It may be a measure of the effectiveness of the search procedure.

Each 'paper patient model' is subdivided into a number of classes (for a description see Chapter V). With the help of these classes comparisons can be made between the styles of the family physician and the general internist. Several hypotheses have been made on this subject.

It was hypothesized that family physicians asked more questions about social background and mental status than did general internists (Smith and McWhinney, 1975; Gerritsma and Smal, 1982). Although family physicians may differ in their search methods, questions about social and emotional troubles constitute a considerable part of the history-taking (Raynes, 1980). Physical examination constitutes a rather variable part of the diagnostic procedure (Raynes, 1980; Hull, 1972). It was hypothesized that general internists spent more time on physical examination than family physicians (Smith and McWhinney, 1975). The same trend could be traced with regard to laboratory and X-ray data. Smith and McWhinney could verify these hypotheses in two of their three simulated patients, while Gerritsma and Smal did not find significant differences.

Our results for the various classes were:

TABLE 19

Variation of search through the different classes of the 'paper patient'

Class	Family physicians %	General internists %
Social background	7.8	3.5
Medical background	9.8	7.0
Medical history	42.9	37.9
Physical examination	31.0	43.7
Laboratory, etc.	8.4	7.9

Family physicians asked more questions about the social background of the patient and performed fewer physical examinations than did general internists.

These results partly corroborate the Smith and McWhinney hypothesis. Obviously, family physicians asked more questions about the social and emotional background of the patient, but history-taking was almost as elaborate for family physicians as for general internists. Physical examination (which was performed by asking specific questions) played a slightly larger part in the diagnostic process of general internists than of family physicians. We found no difference for the laboratory and X-ray class. However, these results should be cautiously interpreted because of the relatively small number of participating internists. To interpret differences in style between these physicians on the basis of class variations seems premature.

On probabilities and (un)certainties

'Decision-making is reducing uncertainty in a problem situation' (Slovic *et al.*, 1977). Initially, before a patient enters the health care system, uncertainty as to the true state of the individual is at a maximum to the people in the system, but by means of a certain set of maneouvres on the part of the health care system and the patient, information is obtained which reduces the uncertainty, to a point, it is hoped, where this information is prescriptive of a course of action (Bohlinger and Ahlers, 1975). Apparently, 'information' is perceived as some kind of evidence which positively guides the problem solver to a solution. However, as we have explained above, all acquired information does not mean positive evidence which can point to a solution, e.g., a diagnosis. Whether a piece of positive evidence, a 'cue', is relevant to a particular (diagnostic) hypothesis depends on the personal conception of the contents of this hypothesis, its symptom-configuration as it is memorized by the physician.

It means that the physician has some prior picture in mind to which a particular datum can be matched and recognised as important to a particular diagnosis (= the prior picture in mind). Any 'cue' presupposes a special relation between the datum and the diagnostic patterns in mind. But when cues reflect the pictures in mind, probability estimates, as chance distributions of symptom-disease relationships, might mirror the personal opinions of physicians and not any objective frequency distribution.

The great variability of probability estimations among physicians can also be attributed to the different kinds of task environment. The family physician as observer of early stage diseases might have a different picture in mind than the clinical specialist who is confronted with the full-blown picture of the disease. Besides, their estimations will clearly be influenced by the numbers of patients they attend to and the frequency of occurrence of particular ailments within their pertinent practice population. Last but not least we have to pose the question whether people can make reliable estimates from observed frequencies. The studies of Kahnemann and Tversky (1972, 1973, 1974) and Fischhoff, Lichtenstein and Slovic (1977, 1978) cast considerable doubts on this capability of human beings.

Our hypothesis, therefore, is that the subjective estimates of prevalence and incidence of diseases by the participating physicians will show a considerable variation.

We asked the participating physicians to estimate the figures of prevalence,[6], incidence,[7] and disease consultation[8] for the particular disease they had diagnosed during the session.

For the family physician in the Netherlands it is quite easy to relate his estimation to a circumscribed population as he, as a result of insurance regulations, attends to a rather stable number of patients, his so-called 'practice population'.

Because the standard deviations grossly surpassed the average of the estimations for each of the rates, any uniformity, any unanimity was found to be non-existent. (A table on this matter is listed in the addendum, Table 33.) Some subsequent observations could be made, such as:

 - the participating physicians obviously related their estimates to recent experiences. Recent calls for extra-uterine pregnancy (as one of the presented cases) made figures jump 20–30 fold;
 - because the investigation took place during the months of February to July, seasonal influences were evident. Figures for bronchitis were highest in the first two months and lowest in the last month.

On a large scale, the variations of the estimates could be related to highly personal, situational and/or seasonal influences, and only partly related to the disease in question. From these figures it may be clear that several assumptions as they are made in clinical decision-making, such as normal probability distributions, tightly clustered values for all patterns in one class, reliable morbidity figures, etc., are not always met in a number of various diseases. And, as Croft (1972) remarks: 'the more grossly the assumptions are violated, the less accurate the diagnoses (made by application of decision analytical approaches) are expected to be'.

An assumption regularly sustained in literature is the relation of these estimates, especially their validity and reliability, to the experience of the physician. It is expected that the more years the physician has spent in real practice the more reliable and valid his estimations. As the years of experience within the group of participating physicians ranged from 0 to 40 years, we could test this assumption on a broad scale. Because the results for all diseases were very similar, we shall present only one graphic table.

The notion of expertise rests an on assumption that medical competence is an innate characteristic of experienced physicians that is generalized across clinical situations. If we assume that more than 10 years of regular clinical practice represents some kind of expertise, we may expect some conformity among the experienced participants regarding the various estimates. Instead we found tremendous differences. Moreover, we found approximately the

---

[6] The number of patients with a certain disease in a circumscribed population (customarily 10,000).
[7] The number of new patients with a certain disease seen by the doctor in a circumscribed time interval (customarily one year).
[8] The number of patients with a certain disease visiting the physician during a circumscribed time interval.

Epidemiological estimates in relation to years of experience for a case of Iron-deficiency anaemia

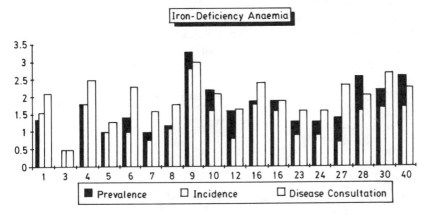

On the horizontal axis the years of experience of the physician is presented. Because of the wide variation of the estimates the vertical axis had to be designed in a logarithmic scale.

same variations among the experienced and the non-(or less) experienced physicians, and between these groups. Any influence of experience or expertise upon the estimates could not be detected.

Decision theory assumes the diagnostic process as a process of sequential steps, each step governed by the pertinent probability estimates of prevalence and symptom-disease relationships. In order to test this theory against the physicians' behaviour, we asked the physicians to identify the degree of weight, or probability, for each hypothesis immediately after its generation. There were two possibilities for (re)adjustment of the subjective probability of a hypothesis. The physicians could adjust their probability estimates in the light of an important cue, and at the same time they were asked to (re)consider their estimation of the previously generated hypotheses in the work-up any time a new hypothesis came to mind. To do that he could enter a mark on an open scale, a horizontal bar. For each hypothesis three bars were available (with more on request): one for the prior probability estimation, one for cue adjustment, and one for the posterior probability. None of the physicians used the possibility of 'cue-adjustment', or the extension of other bars. They all made their estimates on the basis of the generation of hypotheses, thus confirming the concept as described in the inductive inference process.

Sometimes a doctor wished to re-establish a hypothesis which he temporarily quitted during the work-up. He introduced the new (old) hypothesis again with its prior probability, which was usually quite different from the prior probability of the same hypothesis he had generated earlier during the course.

We defined the ultimate point of the diagnostic process in the inductive strategy as a maximization of the disease probability and a minimization of uncertainty. This idea is based on the assumption that the probability estimate expresses a degree of reasonable belief, which leads the doctor to the conviction of being on the right track. This idea is sustained by the figures, although the increase of chance estimates was less than we expected. On average probability figures rose from 0.44 to 0.74. High standard deviations indicate that variance is rather high (see Table 34 Addendum). The variance is presented in the next figure in which the wide variation of the prior probabilities (broken line) as well as the posterior probabilities (solid line) is shown.

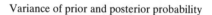

Variance of prior and posterior probability

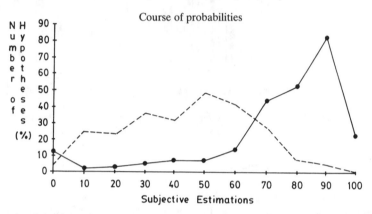

The broad and shallow curve of the prior probabilities reflects the wide variability of the primary hypotheses. From this figure we derive the suggestion that the end of the diagnostic process is partly characterized by a maximization of the subjectively estimated probability to the final hypothesis.

A distinction has been made between doctors who introduced their prior probability on the low side (possibly lower prevalence/incidence rates) and those who introduced high rates. At the end of the work-up nearly all (more than 85%) doctors scored on approximately the same level.

The rate of increase between the first and last probability estimation ranged between 12% and 136% depending on the case. The lowest increase was found in the dermatological case (case 3) and the highest in the endocrinological case (case 6). On average the rate of increase between first and last hypothesis probability estimate was 72%.

It is our opinion that these estimations mainly reflect the physician's confidence in finding a solution for the presented case. Solutions arise during the diagnostic process. The physician conceives it as his task to find that particular solution that can satisfy his own quality standards (and perhaps those of the patient). Probability estimates cannot be viewed as quantitative data in information processing, but must be seen as mirroring the physician's feelings in searching for his way through the problem-solving process.

More or less parallel with the rise (or fall) of confidence in the hypotheses is the physician's confidence in the problem-solving process itself. The values for this latter type of confidence are called the uncertainty estimates. They express the estimation of one's own clinical competence to solve a particular problem.

The values are expressions of one's subjective, emotional feelings of (un)certainty at a given phase of the process. These values were measured in the same manner as the previous (probability) ones: giving an estimation by means of entering a mark on an open bar. In contrast with the probability estimates, people preferred to draw their lines of (un)certainty on a vertical bar, moving upwards with the rise of certainty and vice versa. The participating physician was urged to express his feelings of (un)certainty at two minutes intervals during the work-up, starting immediately after listening to the patient's complaint.

So our first step was to calculate the mean values of the certainty estimate in the successive time score for each of the various subtypes of inductive reasoning. We hoped that the point of onset and the slope of the curve would tell us something about the behaviour of the physicians applying successive methods. The results of this exercise are shown in the next figure (Table 30 Addendum).

Curves of certainty estimates per subtype of inductive reasoning

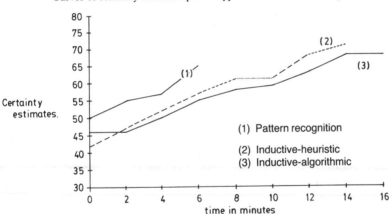

All curves show a gradual progression to a maximum.

These curves would seem to sustain the ideas of Simon's Satisficing theory (see Chapter IV). The curves indicate that, on average, physicians tend to strive for a suboptimal solution which satisfies their adjusted aspiration level. This level is, we presume, largely determined by practice experience. It may be the level of people who know that the optimum is beyond reach but who are happy to live with goals that partly meets their demands with the amount of effort that permits them to survive in a difficult task environment.

The curves also tell us that complete certainty is not a general feeling in clinical practice, because there is no absolute proof of the hypothesis nor is there a single and only explanation for the observed evidence.

The (un)certainty estimates when matched with the various patient cases did not reveal problem-orientation. The (un)certainty estimates show a heterogeneous picture, as could be expected from the notations of the physicians' personal feelings.

Expectations and confidence play a mysterious game. (Un)certainty estimates fluctuated greatly during the session and during each work-up. Highly
confident physicians sometimes fall into despair upon failing to see any solution. Uncertain doctors sometimes welcomed one tiny piece of information
upon which they, very confidently, then built a complete diagnostic construction. We do not and we cannot extract the personal feelings and emotions from
these interacting figures and values. But we have seen people slaving away,
perspiring, we have seen them happy and desperate, drifting from one end of
the certainty scale to the other. We have seen them pleading and shouting to
the 'patient' (the poor simulator), but also begging and advising with all the
conviction they possessed. They addressed the young (male) simulator as
'madam', seriously inquiring about her marriage, her experience in childbirth;
they argued with the 'patient', they sent him away with an advisory list to be
filled in by next week or else. . .! In short, we have seen physicians at work,
with all their emotions and feelings, their hesitations and uncertainties. It was
a tremendous experience. But all these things cannot be caught in figures,
values, curves or statistics. And perhaps so much the better. The human being
is so complex and so unique that dismembering that being into small parts
would deprive him of all his charm.

On patient management and therapy

As we discussed in Chapter I, patient-management and decision-making on
treatment are logical consequences of the diagnostic/prognostic process.
When the disease entity has been established and the natural course of the
disease is known, we can prescribe the pertinent kind of treatment in order to
curve this natural course to a more favourable outcome. The more the natural
course is curved towards a (presumed) favourable outcome within a minimal
time schedule the greater the success. Unfortunately, as disease-entities are
usually ill-defined, natural courses of diseases are generally unknown. We
have often no knowledge of natural courses of diseases as there is no possibility
to study them. To deprive patients of any form of treatment in order to gain
scientific knowledge about the natural courses of disease would be unethical.
So physicians, indeed the whole medical world, is kept in a quandary. In order
to decide upon an efficient treatment we have to know the natural course of a
disease, but we cannot know this because we have to administer some kind of
treatment for ethical, humanitarian, social, psychological, etc., reasons.

The excessive attention in the medical world to treatment cannot be attributed to profound and sincere deliberation, but must be attributed to this
conflict. Most therapies must be conceived as actions to alleviate the patients'
sufferings, leaving recovery to nature and chance.

Physicians, apparently, treat this part of the medical process in a Cinderella-
like way. On average, less than one minute of attention is given to this subject
once a diagnosis is arrived at. In contrast with the patients' views on the
physician's professional activities, the decision maker himself apparently considers it as a minor task. Nevertheless, in that minute a decision is made with

sometimes far-reaching consequences to patients and physicians. We cannot accept this observation as explanatory of physicians' actions. As this finding is a general feature of all physicians' decision-making processes, we propose another explanation. It is our opinion, that the partition of the problem-solving and decision-making clinical process into diagnostic and a therapeutic parts is an artificial one. We hypothesize that within the diagnostic process, as it were, the therapy has already been decided upon. It may be viewed as putting a full stop at the end of a sentence. From this viewpoint each therapy and treatment can only be understood within the context of the whole medical process. It is therefore not this one minute that counts but the preceding process. We shall return to this subject in the next section.

As described in Chapter V, we asked the participants to establish the most appropriate treatment after they had arrived at a diagnosis. This treatment section contains two facets: a facet of involving choosing the action, the direction of treatment, the management of the disease process (e.g., dietary treatment, drugs, physiotherapy, referral to a clinical specialist); and a facet involving specification of the treatment (the medication).

The time involved in making the diagnosis can easily be observed by the simulator as well as from the protocols in the study. The difference between this 'diagnostic' time and the completion of the process was called 'therapy time'. We found on average a 'therapy time' of 1.44 minutes; 128 cases within one minute, 125 between one and two minutes.

Within these one or two minutes the physician performed several tasks among which were:
- informing the patient about the disease;
- deciding upon patient management (drug treatment, medical or hygienic advice, dietary recommendations, referral, consultation, etc.);
- writing a prescription;
- writing a referral note for his colleague specialist;
- informing the patient about the treatment and management.

It is hard to believe that these tasks can be accomplished within this time-scale. In our opinion, this can only be explained by a combination of a well-rehearsed routine and experience. Solutions must lie under the surface to account for this fast retrieval from memory. Furthermore, we suppose that the physicians dwels on treatments and solutions before a final diagnostic decision is made. Indeed, a final decision may even be influenced by the solution already in mind. A definite answer cannot be provided from our material.

Variation across the cases could not be detected. The same can be said about the 'therapy time' as matched to the subtypes of inductive reasoning (see Table 36 Addendum). Quick decisions seem to be an innate characteristic of physicians' behaviour in clinical decision-making. However, the uniformity of swiftness of decision-making does not imply a uniformity of the contents of those decisions. Leaving aside those cases in which a referral to a hospital is inevitable (like myocardial infarction, extra-uterine pregnancy), the general picture is as diverse as it is in symptoms-variance of diagnoses. As we coded all kinds of actions, referrals, and treatment in the 'paper patient' (see Chapter V) we could easily trace and categorize these elements. Consensus of opinion on patient-management could only be discovered in the cases of gall-stones (88% referral to a specialist), and asthmatic bronchitis (100% drug treatment by the family physician). However, on a more detailed level inconsistency governs. For the gall-stone case 50% of the referred patients were sent to an internist, the other 50% to a surgeon. In the case of asthmatic bronchitis nine different categories (!) of drugs were prescribed (by 21 physicians), totalling more than 70 various specified drugs (see Table 37 Addendum).

In the remaining four cases inconsistency dominates the picture, partly because physicians arrived at different diagnoses; yet but even within the group of homonymous diagnoses diversification remains.

Surveying the cases, we get the impression that most of the actions and prescriptions are very personal conceptions. The prescriptions are mainly symptom-oriented instead of cause-related therapy. Most prescribed drugs are 'broad-spectrum' drugs: drugs acting on various domains and causes. For instance, corticotropines are outstanding suppressors of allergic reactions, but they act on a wide range of bodily functions as well. Broad-spectrum antibiotics prescribed in the case of asthmatic bronchitis may be excellent medicaments but by their nature hardly specific. Not only do they attack the bacterial invaders in the lungs but residential bacteria as well.

The personal appreciation and interpretation of the various diseases and their symptoms seems to lead to the variety of drugs. This, in its turn, is consistent with the philosophical backgrounds of inductivism.

On diagnostic gradation

As we discussed in the section On symptoms and diagnoses in this Chapter, the meaning, i.e., the decomposed contents, of a particular diagnosis can vary from person to person. Besides, inconsistency of nomenclature was found to exist among similar symptom-configurations. In case 3 (dermatological case) seven different names were given to an approximately equal configuration of symptoms; in case 7 (respiratory case) eight different names were assigned to a similar pattern. In a number of samples from actual clinical situations we obtained the same results. The degree of variation creates a serious obstacle for meaningful comparisons among physicians, for example, in medical audits, nor can these data be used for the processing of data for statistical applications. Physicians' judgements vary too much for valid analysis.

We are interested in the question whether physicians, given a uniform patient case, would come to the same conclusions. This question was approached in the following way.

Because of the nature of the study we cannot claim one type of diagnosis as correct, and at the same time proclaim another judgement as incorrect. In this study we have to obsever only gradations between agreement on one name of a disease and the lack of any common denominator. For practical reasons we chose four stages of gradation.

(1) one joint name of a disease;

(2) (various) names of diseases belonging to the same organ system;
(3) (various) names of diseases belonging to an adjacent organ system;
(4) (various) names of diseases not belonging to the organ system mentioned in (2) and (3) and having less than 25% of the symptoms mentioned in (1) in common.

We matched this diagnostic gradation to a number of variables, which we have already met in the preceding sections. Some of them are directly related to the inference processes, others are related to states of knowledge of the participating physicians. The former items concern the relation to the cases (problem orientation), to the strategies, and to the consistency of the relationship between diagnoses and treatments. The latter variables concern the physicians' experience and the amount of continuing education.

TABLE 20

Diagnostic gradation and case dependency

Patient case	1		2		3		4		5		6		7		8	
	No.	%	No.	%	No.	%	No.	%	No.	%	No.	%	No.	%	No.	%
Diagn. gradat.																
1	20	65	10	32	9	27	24	73	21	64	27	84	13	43	12	40
2	9	29	14	45	18	55	1	3	9	27	–	–	12	40	11	37
3	1	3	4	13	5	15	7	21	2	6	–	–	4	13	–	–
4	1	3	3	10	1	3	1	3	1	3	5	16	1	3	7	23
Total	31	100	31	100	33	100	33	100	33	100	32	100	30	100	30	100

Focusing on diagnostic gradation (types of corresponding diagnoses or clusters of symptoms) we can see a great variability of the results among the various cases.

With regard to the problem-orientation, the variability of the outcomes of the problem-solving activities can be easily predicted. As we introduced some structure into this variability (diagnostic graduation) we were interested in the degree of variability and the distribution of the various outcomes over the four gradations. The next table shows the results of this relationship.

The variations of diagnostic gradation for the various cases seem rather large. However, we have to realize that uniformity of medical terminology is not one of the stronger points in medical knowledge. It is quite plausible that different physicians use different diagnostic names for the same disease depending on their medical education and referential framework in which they operate. If we assume a diagnostic gradation 2 as a near correct diagnosis (ultimately within the pathology of the correct organ system), the variation may be less than expected. Taking gradation 1 and 2 together the consensus of opinion about a disease ranges between 76% and 94%. The problem remains, of course, that we cannot know what diagnoses, defined as a particular symptom-configuration, actually belong to one specified entity. Diseases have abstract names which perfectly hide their concrete contents. Communicating in the language of disease nomenclature is like exchanging objects in the dark. You may never be quite sure about the thing you have laid a hand on.

The matching of the various subtypes of the inductive reasoning does not present striking differences with regard to the gradation.

As for the question which method scores highest for the diagnostic gradations 1 and 2 the algorithmic mode scores slightly better than the others {71 to 58 (P-R) and 45 (Heur.)}. Although being basically the same (inductive) the algorithmic method has less tendency to overlook possible cues which can lead to more accurate hypotheses. As the algorithmic method was employed predominantly by the general internists, evidently the outcome for the diagnostic gradations 1 and 2 must be slightly better for internists than for family physicians. Taking these gradations together the internists scored 96% against the family physicians 82%. For diagnostic gradation 1 the results were respectively 67% and 46%. These findings do not imply a better diagnostic procedure on the part of the internists. It may be possible that, as we expect, medical terminology among general internists is more uniform than among family physicians. This latter category of doctor is, as a matter of task environment, confronted with a much broader variety of diseases, illnesses and social troubles.

TABLE 21

Distribution of types of strategy versus diagnostic gradation

Strategy	Patt. recogn.		Induct. heur.		Induct. algor.		Total
	row%	col%	row%	col%	row%	col%	
Diagn. gradat.							
1	18.8[a]	24.5	68.0	23	13.2	38	100
2	26.6	33.5	62.7	22	11.2	33	100
3	17.4	22.2	82.6	29	–	–	100
4	15.0	19.8	75.0	26	10.0	29	100
Total		100		100		100	

[a] The number of records is standardized for each of the variables.

We tried to create a similar gradation system for the therapy part of the medical process. Here again we lack a more or less generally accepted nomenclature. There is no general agreement about optimal treatment; one can expect to find only some individual recommendation and personal preference. A joint denominator on therapy cannot easily be found. To bypass this obstacle we used a book in the possession of all physicians, because it was sent to them free of charge. It is the counterpart of a textbook known in the U.S.A. as 'Current Medical Diagnosis and Treatment', and revised, translated and published in the Netherlands in 1983. For each disease a concise treatment recommendation is advised. Our gradation for therapy runs as follows:

(a) the advice in the book is followed completely or at least for three-

quarters of the advised remedies;
  (b) half or more of the recommendations for that particular disease are followed;
  (c) less than half of the advised remedies are prescribed;
  (d) neither a, b, or c can be applied.

We are aware of the vulnerability of this system, but at least it will give some indication, some awareness of the physician's behaviour. Within this context we shall give some figures matching the diagnostic gradation with its therapeutic counterpart.

The figures in Table 22 represent the number of records to which both a diagnostic gradation and a therapeutic gradation pertains. To test the consistency between these two variables, we calculated for each cell the standardized predicted values from the totals of each class of gradation where the values follow the relative composition of these totals. It is calculated as the total of a certain diagnostic class multiplied by the total of the applicable therapeutic gradation class divided by the total number of records.

TABLE 22

Distribution and consistency for the variables: diagnostic and therapeutic gradation

Diagnostic gradation	1		2		3		4		Total
Therap. gradation	Real	Exp	Real	Exp	Real	Exp	Real	Exp	
a	88	60	26	44	9	11	3	10	126
b	27	48	53	36	12	9	10	8	102
c	6	10	9	7	1	2	5	2	21
d	–	2	1	1	1	–	2	–	4
Total	121		89		23		20		253

Diagnostic consensus and therapeutic conformity seem to coincide. The less diagnostic consensus the less therapeutic conformity is to be found. The question of the consistency between these two variables is answered by the calculation of the expected values for each box of this cross-table. The deviations to the real figures indicate a considerable consistency between the variables.
REAL = real values as were found in the investigation.
EXP = values as expected from calculation (explanation in text).

E.g., for the upper left hand cell (1a) the calculation is:

    $121 \times 126 / 253$

and for cell 2b

    $89 \times 102 / 253$

The more the real value differs from the expected value the more consistency has to be assumed.

The most striking phenomenon in this table is, in my opinion, that the more uniform the diagnosis, the more consensus we can find on the part of the therapy. The highest gradations from both sides match at 72%, all other gradations are strikingly lower. The second stage of both gradations scores 60% and decreases relatively with (decreasing) diagnostic gradation. The lower gradation on the diagnostic side also scores remarkably low in the therapeutic part. Apparently, diagnostic and therapeutic uniformity and consensus parallel each other. This aspect deserves great attention. As we have mentioned before, the action of management and treatment cannot be viewed as separate parts of the medical process. Both are parts of the same process and the same strategy.

It is widely assumed that experience in clinical practice contributes largely to clinical competence. We expect experience to be a trend towards increasing diagnostic skills. We defined 'experience' as the number of years actually spent practising in clinical health care. We distinguished three groups: group 1, 0–5 years of practice; group 2, 6–20 years; and group 3, more than twenty years. The results of the matching of diagnostic gradation and experience are shown in the next table.

TABLE 23

Physicians' experience versus diagnostic gradation

Experience groups 0–5 years			6–20 years		more than 20 years	
Diagnostic gradation	No.	%	No.	%	No.	%
1	13	48	87	51	21	38
2	7	26	59	35	23	41
3	3	11	13	8	7	13
4	4	15	11	6	5	9
Total	27	100	170	100	56	100

Consistency of diagnostic nomenclature among physicians does not necessarily increase with advanced experience.

Increasing experience does not contribute to the consistency of nomenclature. Even if we add diagnostic gradation 1 and 2 (and circumvent the problem of medical terminology) any indication of a substantial increase in diagnostic skills will be sought in vain. Apparently, 'experience' has a far more complex impact on medical knowledge or its application than was thought.

Along a similar line of thought we had assumed that a varying amount of continuing education would affect the diagnostic gradation. From an inquiry among the participants of the investigation we learned that with regard to continuing education three groups could be distinguished: a group that spent less than 9.2 days per 2 years on official courses; a group of more than 9.2 days/2 years; a group following no formal courses. The result of the matching is shown in the following table.

TABLE 24

Diagnostic gradation versus continuing education

Diagnostic gradation	Continuing education[b]					
	Less than 9.2 days		More than 9.2 days		No courses	
	No.	%	No.	%	No.	%
1	42[a]	48	61	48	18	43
2	31	38	42	33	16	38
3	6	8	13	10	4	9.5
4	4	6	12	9	4	9.5
Total	83	100	128	100	42	100

[a] Number of records = number of solved 'patients'.
[b] Continuing education refers to official courses within a two-year period.

From this table it follows that whatever amount of continuing education is attended (or not), improved consensus of diagnostic nomenclature does not automatically result.

Apparently, consensus of diagnostics does not improve as a result of continuing education. We can think of several explanations:
  (a) courses do not focus on diagnostic procedures;
  (b) courses are more concerned with new developments in medicine;
  (c) courses have not been validated towards routine practice situations.
We cannot elaborate on this from our material. Further studies in this field may be recommended.

On experience and consequences

It is widely believed that experience improves the clinical competence and the inference qualities of physicians. The notion of expertise rests on the presumption that diagnostic skill is an innate trait of experienced physicians that is generalized across clinical situations. However, Elstein and colleagues (1978) failed to demonstrate any difference between a group of 17 judged by their peers to be highly proficient diagnosticians ('criterial group') and another group of seven who were not so nominated ('non-criterial group'). These findings do not support the widespread belief that designation of expertise by medical peers is well-founded and well-validated (McGaghie, 1980). It also questions the expertise itself. According to Brehmer (1980), improvement of clinical competence and expertise on the basis of clinical experience is founded on an incorrect understanding of the nature of experience. Indeed, scrutinizing this notion leads to a more pessimistic view about people's ability to learn from experience (see also Goldberg, 1968).

In this paragraph we shall match some of the above-mentioned variables to the experience of the participants. The experience is expressed in terms of years in medical practice, in day-to-day service in health care. In the section on probability and (un)certainty we indicated that any trend in experience-related estimation for prevalence, incidence and disease consultation values could not be detected.

In this section we split the group of participants into three compartments: the younger, expected to be the non-experienced group of physicians with a practice experience between 0 and 5 years, a middle group with 6 to 20 years in practice, and a group of physicians with more than 20 years in health care service. These groups represent respectively 11, 67 and 22 percent of the total of 253 records (which is in congruency with the distribution of physicians in the actual population of physicians).

When experience plays a part in gaining insight, knowledge or competence in medical problem-solving skils we may expect a more-or-less linear trend across the various variables. In the following tables we shall present a number of these variables matched with the three 'experience groups'.

One of the assumptions made in literature (e.g., de Dombal, 1973) is that the more senior the doctor, the more relevant information is sought in the least number of questions. As described in the first section of this Chapter we defined a relevancy factor from the symptoms which could be allocated to a hypothesis and those which could not.

The symptoms which could be attributed to a particular hypothesis were called hypothesis prerelated symptoms (HPS) and the hypothesis related symptoms (HRS). These symptoms contrast with those which could not be attributed to these (or other) hypotheses, namely, non-hypothesis-related symptoms (NHRS). The relevancy factor could thus be delineated as

$$\frac{HPS + HRS}{HPS + HRS + NHRS} \times 100.$$

The more relevant to a particular hypothesis were the symptoms asked the higher the factor. Confirmation of the assumption means that we may expect an upward tendency of the relevancy factor with increasing experience. The second part of the suggestion predicts a downward tendency of the number of questions asked with increasing experience.

TABLE 25

Physicians' experience versus relevancy factor

Experience groups	Relevancy factor
0–5 years	61.2
6–20 years	65.5
> 20 years	68.5

The assumption that more experience leads to the acquisition of more relevant information can scarcely be sustained when matched with the relevancy factor.

The first part of the hypothesis seems to be slightly corroborated. The second part, however, does not sustain the assumption. In fact, significant

TABLE 26

Physicians' experience versus mean number of questions

Experience groups	Number of questions	St. dev.
0–5 years	32.04	11.08
6–20 years	43.49	21.31
> 20 years	31.66	15.13

The thought that more experienced physicians ask fewer questions (but more relevant ones) than their younger colleagues cannot be confirmed by these figures.

differences with respect to the total number of questions between the three groups could not be traced.[9]

To test the possibility that the 'oldest' group adopted a more leisurely time-schedule, we also matched the groups with the mean total time used for solving a patient case.

Again we could find no differences between the groups with regard to time spent.

Another question is whether more experienced physicians are more elaborate in their generation of hypotheses. In the literature different opinions are found. Some authors believe the experts to be more specific in their work-up with correspondingly fewer hypotheses, while others assume a different attitude. Our results are presented in the next table.

TABLE 27

Physicians' experience versus mean total time

Experience groups	Total time (mean)	St. dev.
0–5 years	11.81	3.75
6–20 years	11.79	6.05
> 20 years	12.08	4.97

Experience does not influence the time needed to solve a patient's problem.

Although differences are small, we may assume that a trend exists indicating that expertise parallels specificity of the work-up. We wondered whether this notion is reflected in the subjective estimates of prior and posterior probabilities of the hypotheses. It may be recalled from section 5 of this Chapter that it was assumed that the prior probability reflected the prevalence (or incidence) rates of the supposed disease, and the posterior probabilities as the adjustment of the prior probability considering the acquired information. It is a widely held belief in primary health care that inexperienced family physicians lack the

[9] As the group with 6–20 years of experience contains the higher number of general internists who predominantly practise the inductive-algorithmic strategy, the number of questions is shifted to a higher level.

TABLE 28

Physicians' experience and the generation of hypotheses

Experience groups	Number of hypotheses (mean values)	St. dev.
0–5 years	3.55	1.65
6–20 years	2.89	1.55
> 20 years	2.79	1.12

From the mean number of hypotheses and the standard deviations we may conclude a slight tendency towards the generation of fewer hypotheses with increasing experience.

knowledge and insight into the frequency distribution of diseases and their symptoms in more or less specified populations. Therefore the problem-solving process of inexperienced or less experienced (family) physicians should be less optimal when compared to their more experienced colleagues.

We matched the figures of prior probability and posterior probability, as they are presented in the section on probability and (un)certainty, with the experience groups.

TABLE 29

Physicians' experience and their estimates of prior and posterior probabilities

Experience group	First probability		Last probability	
	Mean	St. dev.	Mean	St. dev.
0–5 years	39.26	24.01	73.26	23.77
6–20 years	47.58	20.24	73.85	25.20
>20 years	36.43	20.31	74.38	22.94

Remarkably, the group of physicians with an experience in medical practice of 6 to 20 years estimated the prior probabilities for their first hypotheses higher than the other groups. On the diagnostic level the posterior probability estimates bring the groups together.

As we have seen in the figure on epidemiological estimates in relation to years of experience (section on Probability and (un)certainty) the values for prior probabilities of the 'youngest' and the 'oldest' groups astonishingly resemble each other, while the 'middle' group takes a different position. With regard to posterior probabilities, only an optimist will observe a tendency towards increasing experience.

Probability estimates, as weighting factors for the hypotheses, sometimes reflect the state of (un)certainty of the physician. Therefore, we matched this variable also with the experience groups.

The more experienced physicians seem to be slightly less certain when confronted with a new problem. However, this may also be an artefact of the investigation. The simulation scenario with video camera might have been more threatening to them than to their younger colleagues, as the latter group

TABLE 30

Physicians' experience and their feelings of uncertainty

Experience groups	First certainty estimate		Last certainty estimate	
	Mean values	St. deviat.	Mean values	St. deviat.
0–5 years	45.44	27.70	61.33	26.34
6–20 years	44.12	29.32	69.59	21.34
>20 years	35.36	27.63	65.32	23.30

Primary uncertainty is highest for the most experienced physicians, although the values for standard deviations make firm conclusions hazardous. The last certainty estimates (on the diagnostic level) are approximately on an even level.

grew accustomed to this equipment during their days in medical school.

With regard to management and treatment one might expect more restraint in the 'older' group towards referral of patients to hospitals and specialists. Their knowledge of and insight into prognosis, courses of illness and the various reactions to drugs are greater than those of their less experienced colleagues. We matched two features of therapeutic action, prescription and referral, with the three experience groups.

Again, any differences between the groups are sought in vain.

We also calculated the distribution of the subtypes of inductive reasoning across the three experience groups.

TABLE 31

Physicians' experience and treatment plans for prescription and referral

Experience groups	Prescription	Referral
0–5 years	48%	52%
6–20 years	49%	51%
>20 years	50%	50%

(The percentages are calculated from the number of the particular actions divided by the total number of solved cases within that particular experience group.)
Differences of conception with regard to patient management between the experience groups are not found.

Apart from the algorithmic mode, marked differences between the experience groups with regard to the employment of the subtypes of inductive reasoning could not be found.

Considering a number of relevant items within the clinical problem-solving process we could trace no effects from clinical experience defined as years in health care practice. This observation is contradictory to most conceptions about experience in the medical world. It underscores the critical views on competence deriving from clinical experience of authors like Brehmer, 1980, Goldberg, 1968, Oskamp, 1965. It does not mean that experience is a negligible factor in human cognition and reasoning, but its contribution is far more

TABLE 32

Physicians' experience and their employment of the strategies

Experience groups	Pattern recognition	Heuristic	Algorithmic	Total
0–5 years	14.9	85.1	–	100
6–20 years	23.3	62.0	14.7	100
>20 years	16.0	78.7	5.3	100

The 'middle' group constitutes the largest group of physicians using the pattern recognition method as well as the algorithmic strategy. This latter observation may be due to the number of general internists included in this group.

complex than a simple linear relationship. It is our opinion that as long as the reasoning process and its outcome bears a (very) personalistic imprint, it cannot contribute to the generalisation of medical knowledge, and cannot, therefore, be submitted to the proof of validity and reliability. For simple algorithms, as for instance in certain tool-handling, a direct relation between experience and performance can be presumed. But when more complicated processes, like medical problem-solving and decision-making are involved, even a very small number of relevant factors might have an indeterminate effect on improved performance. These effects, however, are difficult to demonstrate and to prove.

Still we need to understand the clinical process in order to describe its components, to comprehend its actions and operations and to make it accessible to education and research. However, the consequences of the inductive approach and the subsequent individualistic character of the physician's knowledge seem to create a nearly surmountable barrier to a better understanding.

Summary

The criteria which were used to characterise the models depicted in Chapter V were compared to the collected material. This consisted of data from 253 patient-cases as solved by 68 physicians: 60 family physicians and 8 general internists. The analysis revealed that only one type of reasoning could be identified: the inductive method. The subtypes of the inductive method add a special accent to the various aspects of this method. The inductive method seems to be the best explanation of the various problems, questions and dilemmas discussed in the previous chapters. The inductive method is a method in which hypotheses are compared and weighed against other hypotheses in order to find the most satisfying one for diagnosis. It means a collection of hypotheses rather than a process of proof. Rejection of hypotheses, therefore, is an infrequent occurrence. It also leads to the mixing of information and to testing data in a circular process.

As the hypotheses stem from memorized disease-pictures, the symptom-configurations of the hypotheses can differ from physician to physician, from day to day. The nomenclature resembles general names as they are used within medical knowledge. However, when decomposing the hypotheses/diagnoses into their constituent symptoms a profound inconsistency among the disease-pictures could be found. There even exists a considerable difference between the memorized picture and the actual data as collected during the work-up of a case.

The efficiency of information acquisition and processing is one of the major topics in the discipline of medical informatics. As the physician/patient encounter assumes an individualistic character it is rather difficult to establish the physician's competence in this respect. To gain insight into the efficiency of the process we created three distinct measures: ratio effectiveness, content effectiveness, and retrieval rate. Decreasing ratio effectiveness during the course of the process might be a factor which contributes to the shutdown of the problem-solving and decision-making process because of diminishing yield of information. The figures for content-effectiveness and retrieval rate suggest that the eliciting of 'positive symptoms' from the patient ('the clinical database') is not the mark of the physician's greatest capabilities.

Next in importance to these factors an increase in the (posterior) probability and a decrease of uncertainty also trigger an end to the diagnostic process in the inductive way of reasoning. the subjective probability estimates by our physician subjects for a number of epidemiological factors relevant to the cases studied showed wide fluctuations. Therefore, we hypothesize that probability estimations by physicians in our study express his/her personal feelings of (un)certainty rather than numeric calculations of frequency.

Annexed to the question of the reliability of probability estimations is the problem of diagnostic inconsistency. Next to incongruency of medical nomenclature inconsistency as to the composing symptoms of a disease description complicates the picture. The reliability of objective probability estimates when they are derived from large clinical data-bases if not corrected for these types of inconsistency must be seriously questioned.

Consensus of opinion about diagnostic entities is difficult to find among doctors. Inconsistency not only seems to be related to the particular case but to the personality of the physician also. It hampers the development of epidemiology as a firm basis for statistical and decision-making purposes. It sets constraints to the analysis of national and international classifications of diseases, and conclusions derived from such an analysis without accurate and precise definition of the medical nomenclature, health care policy and management must continue to be based on weak foundations.

An individualistic prespective probably also extends to the patient management and treatment part of the clinical process. Wide variability in choices of actions and prescriptions are the rule rather than the exception. Because the decision on a treatment is reached within 1-2 minutes, we hypothesized that making a choice of a clinical action actually takes place during the diagnostic phase of the process. We cannot avoid the impression that the availability of a particular solution strongly influences the ultimate choice in the therapeutic phase of the process.

Experienced doctors often have a small number of highly efficient solutions at hand; solutions which they know have a reasonable chance of success in a high percentage of cases. However, the circular reasoning of inductive inference leads the doctor to believe in the effectiveness of his solution without necessarily having any proof of this assumption. 'Experience' creates the probability estimates of success. These estimates are based on memorized cases in the near past, almost all of which are linked with favourable results.

In our material we could not detect any effect of experience on a number of factors relevant to clinical processes. If there is any effect of experience on clinical competence, its relationship is a very complex one and as yet undiscovered.

TABLE 33

Prevalence, incidence, disease-consultation rate estimates for 8 disease-entities

Disease	Prevalence[a]		Incidence		Disease consultation	
	Mean	St. dev.	Mean	St. dev.	Mean	St. dev.
Myoc. inf.	2.21	4.69	48.32	23.95	114.32	128.75
Ischial.	133.80	203.77	460.30	981.96	707.60	1070.04
Gall	147.61	247.10	21.72	17.23	83.72	90.70
Hyperth.	50.63	52.38	12.33	17.50	90.67	166.99
Bronch.	337.88	645.84	1287.38	1372.84	2918.63	3485.97
E.u.pr.	3.05	10.89	8.38	6.26	9.67	9.45
Anaemia	206.35	510.83	64.35	165.41	194.90	254.77

[a] The figures are standardized for a population of 10,000.

TABLE 34

From the first (hypothesis) probability estimate to the last (hypothesis) probability

Increase of probability estimates per strategy.

Strategy	First probability		Last probability		Increase
	Mean value	St. dev.	Mean value	St. dev.	
Patt. recogn.	51.80	19.68	77.40	24.49	33.63
Induct. heurist.	41.28	21.67	73.74	23.94	32.46
Induct. algorithm.	47.86	15.92	69.96	28.11	22.10
Mean total	44.22	21.16	73.91	24.47	29.69

(Figures are given in percentages.)
The estimates represent the weights which are given to a particular hypothesis. This weight is an expression of the physician's confidence of being on the right track towards a solution. Across the various hypotheses which are generated in the course of the solution these weights follow the line of the physician's search and reasoning. These estimates give us indications about the physician's problem-solving behaviour, not precise calculations.

TABLE 35

Certainty estimates per strategy (mean values)

Strategy	First certainty estimate	Last certainty estimate
Pattern recognition	48.9	67.4
Inductive-heuristic	41.1	67.0
Inductive-algorithm.	44.6	70.3

The boldness of the physicians employing the pattern recognition method per se contrasts with the more or less uniformly lower first certainty estimates of the other strategies. In the end they all come together.

TABLE 36

'Therapy time' per strategy

Strategy	Time until diagnosis mean values	Total time mean values	Therapy time mean values
Pattern recognit.	7.96	9.41	1.45
Induct.-heurist.	10.70	12.14	1.44
Induct.-algorith.	20.08	21.54	1.46

The differences between the time periods for the total work-up must be exclusively attributed to the diagnostic part. For all three strategies 'therapy time' remains the same.

TABLE 37

Prescriptions for a case of asthmatic bronchitis

Name medicament-group	Number	%
Antibiotics: tetracyclines	9	19
Expectorans/mucolyticum	9	19
Antibiotic: broad spectrum penicillines	8	17
Spasmolytics: xanthine-derivatives	5	11
Adrenergica: sympathicomimetics	5	11
Emollientia	4	9
Cough depressing drugs	3	6
Corticotropines	2	4
Antihistaminics	2	4

Nine different groups of medicaments have been prescribed for the cases of asthmatic bronchitis. These nine groups of medicaments stand for 50 *different* drugs.

Chapter VII

Reflections, conclusions, consequences

> The field of genuine success: correct prediction from theory.

Introduction

We shall again face the questions posed in the Introduction and, try to find some answers. Do patients benefit from their doctor's advice? Do physicians know what they are doing? How do we know what the best advice is? Are the methods that doctors use in medical practice the most appropriate, valid, reliable, and efficient ones? Do physicians' methods reach the standards of present-day conceptions of science? Is medicine an art or a science?

We suggested that in order to answer the first five questions the answer to the last one was of crucial importance. As art is subjective, implicit, irreproducible, and incapable of precise analysis, any measurement is doomed to failure. But without precise measurement we are unable to answer the posed questions. Without these answers we remain ignorant about the effectiveness and efficiency of health care as provided by clinical medicine.

Science can not only provide these answers but can also be explanatory of the various questions and problems we meet and have met in clinical medicine. But here we are struck by the ambivalence of the term 'science'. Science does not seem to be that monolithic structure that most people assume it to be. Science is sometimes thought of as some kind of theorizing about far away concepts; science is understood to be some shrewd and astute way of looking for the truth; science is sometimes alleged to be a kind of 'eureka' occurrence; it is supposed to represent the true and only wisdom. But science is also taken as a belief, as philosophying about some better way of living, or leading to the one and only universal Truth. Science is supposed to provide creative devices and statistics which will guide and destine our future and fate.

Obviously we are in need of some definition, or more appropriately, some statement about 'science'; at least the way I see 'science' within the context of this book. As is the case with most abstract names, the term 'science' denotes various concrete collections of different concrete things. There are scientific theories, explaining parts of the knowledge contained within a particular (scientific) discipline; there are hypotheses inviting scientists to test them in order to come nearer to satisfactory explanations, or even the truth; there are methods of ascertaining the truth of a scientific hypothesis, or methods alleging the hypothesis to be probable or unacceptable.

According to Braithwaite (1968) 'the function of a science (. .) is to establish general laws covering the behaviour of empirical events, or objects with which the science in question is concerned'. This characterization emphasizes its concern with empirical phenomena, together with its function in expanding the knowledge of the laws concerning these phenomena (Forstrom, 1977). This conception includes the study and understanding of disease processes and the methodology by which to diagnose, to treat and to prevent these diseases. It encompasses the firm construction of a consistent and reliable knowledge base as well as the methodology pertinent to this construction.

The founders of the subject of scientific methodology, like Plato, Aristotle, Bacon, Descartes, Kant, Mill, etc. believed in some method of discovering scientific truth. In later days more skeptical methodologists no longer believed that it was possible to find one universal law of Nature that would explain everything, but in discovering a theory which, at least temporarily, might be explanatory of a number of phenomena. The conceptions held by the philosophers and methodologists about the ways to reach such reliable and explanatory theories differed at certain fundamental points. These differences can be condensed into two schools: a school of inductive methodology, and a school of deductive reasoning. Both schools have had their fervent adherents to the present days. As we discussed in Chapter II we adopted the deductive way of reasoning as being the scientific standard of explanation. Although inductive reasoning is the far more common method of inference in research as well as in daily life, its consequences lead, even must lead, to individualistic beliefs and standpoints, which does not contribute to a consistent field of knowledge. Our hypothesis is that non-logical inference methods lead to non-logical knowledge, which in turn contributes to non-logical reasoning, and so on.

For the purposes of the investigation we designed two models which could substitute for clinical reasoning: a deductive and an inductive one. We assumed these models to be explanatory of the problem-solving and decision-making processes of practising physicians. We expected the models to be explicative of a number of questions which arose in the study. We assumed these models to be invariant in the variable circumstances that can be encountered in clinical situations. The criteria resulting from these models could enable identification of the methods from the observed evidence. These models enabled us to find some answers to the original questions of the study:
– how do physicians solve problems?
– how do physicians make their decisions?
– do they employ special methods or strategies in order to reach a solution or decision?
– are these methods related to the structure of medical knowledge?
– can this structure be specified in terms of a logical schema of statements and of classes of statements?

Only one of the models appeared to be invariably present among the 253 problem-solving and decision-making processes of the 68 physicians. The question whether these 253 cases and 68 physicians represent the clinical world cannot be definitely answered from the material. The study refutes a deductive inference process as a unique, or dominant, method of problem-solving in clinical medicine. Although we designed two models, the remaining one does not necessarily represent the truth. This model, the inductive one, is strongly supported by critical evidence; it successfully predicted certain outcomes and consequences. It could clarify and explain a number of features of the clinical reasoning process. The model would suggest further thorough investigation into that particular and peculiar world of physicians' thinking in clinical medicine.

The inductive method in medicine

Almost everybody believes in induction. It is the strong belief that we can by sheer force of logic predict from a single event the verisimilitude of similar events to come. Inductive inference (and judgement) carries the conviction of prediction and truth. To generalize from the particular it is believed that a particular event will present itself in future on many more occasions and in approximately equal form. We believe the prediction to be true because we believe the inference and the evidence upon which the judgement rests to be true. The evidence for the inductive statement stems from successful past applications of induction. The theory of induction holds that we experience many things of a similar kind. It creates a 'habit of mind' which makes us believe that we will see more things of the same kind. Then, when we have seen five white swans, we believe the sixth will be white too. This means that our belief in the inductive reasoning is strengthened when we see many similar things. But how do we know that the things that we encounter are really similar and instances of the same phenomenon? If we still continue to feel that there is some consistent relation between our beliefs and the factual evidence present-ed to us, we must regard this reasoning (with Hume) as a mere habit without acknowledging any justification of the convictions expressed by the habit.

The function of inductive reasoning is not to discover something new, but to establish familiarity with something previously discovered. Its function is not to make us conscious of a new problem but to eliminate as far as possible all variant and disturbing factors in order to concentrate on the subject which is familiar to us.

Problem-solving in an inductive way, therefore, is a much more practical approach than the deductive method. For instance, by selecting a response which is known by experience to be 'positive' we can discard many more diagnostic hypotheses than we could if we were to consider a 'negative' response (Blois, 1980). By an early formulation of a small number of diag-nostic hypotheses, doctors can limit the search area of the clinical entities. This restriction enables them to concentrate on a particular hypothesis(es) and on communication with the patient. It saves time and the percentage of hitting the 'right' answer is, seen from the experiential viewpoint of the doctor, rather high. Indeed, the notion of accidentally hitting on specific and/or explanatory cues or hypotheses when following some personally appreciated, heuristic steps and rules (clinical intuition), the 'art-form' of medicine, is so widespread that it is assumed to be *the* method of choice in dealing with patient's problems.

However, an impairment is that we cannot know whether these intuitive flashes of insight are casual & frequent, whether they lead to optimal decisions or not, or whether they serve the purpose of enhancing the physician's competence.

Frequently, physicians take diagnoses for granted more or less unconsciously, and therefore uncritically. These uncritically accepted diagnoses are the strongest reason to hold the diagnosis to be true. For in inductive reasoning we believe in the diagnosis, we believe in the observed evidence which supports the diagnosis, and we belief in the similarity of the presented case with one or more cases in the past. We believe in regularities because without this conviction we are cast into the uncertainties of chaos. As we quoted earlier, 'the last thing anyone would likely to entertain is a state of uncertainty'. In our opinion, this is one of the main reasons for adopting and maintaining the inductive inference method as the method of choice for solving problems in daily life.

People regularly infer general statements from particular elements or single observations. They often reduce complicated questions to comprehensible sizes and then jump to conclusions. They often make general conclusions from special memorized events or specific experiences and repeat them as valuable advice to their friends and relatives. They estimate chances from single perceptions and when the outcome is flawed they invent new and different arguments to support a general statement sometimes opposed to the former one. Inductive reasoning can be observed every day in daily life, on television, in newspapers, in politics, etc. We are so accustomed to this type of reasoning that it passes without notice. It can be viewed as an innate trait of the human being.

However, when knowledge stems from memorized events and personal perceptions of occurrences, all knowledge becomes knowledge of what is going on in our own minds. The world becomes the totality of my ideas, of my dreams. All measurement is related to this world. When hypotheses are tested against other hypotheses, they are weighed according to my own personal standards. Subjective estimates become the expression of personal feelings, the feelings of expectation, confidence, or uncertainty, instead of being rationally deduced statistics. They express the person's beliefs or his doubts which may be aroused by certain assertions or conjectures. Testing of hypotheses in the inductive method is comparing the physician's private convictions to the standards of his own world.

The validity of the outcome is based upon the proportion of former favourite experiences which led to conclusions which were true for the subject. Therefore, a medical diagnosis can only be regarded as a very special personal statement containing a personal opinion and prediction. Questioning this statement is to question the person. The physician has committed himself to his judgement. The reflective physician is then caught in an insoluble conflict between a demand for impersonality which would discredit all commitments (to the judgement) and an urge to make up his mind which drives him to recommit himself (Polanyi, 1958).

Success was achieved to the extent that we ascertained a mode of problem-solving consistent across the spectrum of physicians, problems and situations. We realize that generalizations from this study may be hazardous. However, the methods and the procedures that physicians employ in solving patients' problems are so strikingly similar and uniform across the various physicians and problems, that as a result we cannot see why the 68 physicians who participated in this study should essentially be different from their colleagues elsewhere. As we argued above a notable characteristic of the medical profession is that its practitioners almost unfailingly recognize each other's troubles, behaviour, and working patterns. This study elucidated these working patterns as components of an explicit method as it is employed in day-to-day practice.

We shall recapitulate and discuss a number of the characteristics of this method.

On the circular process

As we discussed in Chapter II, and modelled in Chapter V, a special feature of inductive inference is its circularity of reasoning. In an explanatory reasoning process a set of statements are arranged in such a way that one of these statements describes the state of affairs to be explained (the explicandum) and the others, the explanatory statements, form the 'explanation' in the narrow sense of the word (the explicans of the explicandum). It will be clear that if the explicans is not known to be true (which is usually the case) there must be independent evidence in its favour, or the explicans must be independently testable. When the explicans is proved by the explicandum a circular reasoning is created, for instance:

> 'Why is this person so pale?' – 'Because he is ill' – 'By what evidence can you support your statement that this person is ill?' – 'Oh, can't you see he is pale? And is that not always the case when people are ill?'

This explanation is found to be unsatisfactory because the only evidence for the explicans stems from the explicandum, thus leading to circularity. The physician is thus conducted towards what he believes to be the truth. The only evidence stems from his own reasoning process which he is convinced is correct. As it is the outcome and not the process that comes to our attention (Miller, 1956), this outcome cannot stand for any true explanation of the observation. However, the true inductivist believes that retrospective analysis of the reasoning process can reveal its flaws or lacunae; that the thinking process is logically accountable and can be logically spelled out. It is precisely in this respect that induction fails to be a true explanation of the state of affairs. Too many restrictions and personal convictions and perceptions are built into the process. For instance, the physician restricts his search deliberately by early hypothesis formulation (illness because of paleness) and collects evidence in support of this hypothesis (paleness because of illness). He short cuts his reasoning process by directing it to the idea in mind of which he is the only proprietor and proof. Testing of the hypothesis and information acquisition are conducted on the same principle, and cannot, therefore, be an independent test for the explicans.

By denoting the symptoms in a way that enabled us to relate the symptoms to the hypotheses we were able to test this circular structure in the practice of clinical reasoning. We defined the process between the generation of two hypotheses as one cycle. Within this cycle both elements, the testing symptoms (related to the formulated hypothesis) and the informative symptoms (related to the following hypothesis) are active at the same level of explanation. Neither 'type' of symptom functions as independent evidence which can be deduced from the presented facts. Instead they act as some coupling element between two hypotheses. This is, according to McLuhan, exactly what people do: coupling ideas to ideas, concepts to concepts, patterns to patterns. This procedure substitutes for human thinking, which is, in his vision, prostituted by an easy message wrapped in tinsel.

As we have discussed in Chapter III the idea of coupling ideas/hypotheses to ideas/hypotheses is in conformity with conceptions about human thinking processes. The recoding procedure organizes the stimulus input into a sequence of chunks, each containing a variable number of informational elements. As a chunk is 'any structure that has become familiar from previous repeated exposure and hence is recognizable as a single unit' (Miller, 1956), a chunk is perfectly reconcilable with a hypothesis in inductive reasoning. Because chunks act as devices to overcome the informational bottleneck of the Short Term Memory, it is easily understood why the operation of coupling hypotheses is a convenient way to avoid intellectual strain and hence contributes to an easy and efficient management in clinical affairs. Therefore, the cycling process from hypothesis to hypothesis, storing hypotheses in an equal level arrangement for weighing them against each other, seems to be a natural trait when seen from the point of view of the thinking processes.

On hypotheses

As we discussed in the previous section, hypotheses play an important role in the problem-solving procedure of the physician. They serve to focus ideas and patterns of attention which conduct the doctor through the process which will eventually lead to a decision. They also function as 'chunks' to transcend the natural mental bottleneck towards our nearly unlimited memory space in Long Term Memory.

Unlike the hypotheses in deductive reasoning, the hypotheses within the inductive strategy are not hierarchically arranged from more general towards detailed levels of specification. There is no logical relationship between the collected hypotheses. It prevents any retracing of the mental steps taken by the physician in order to solve the problem. Consequently, hypotheses in inductive reasoning do not represent a number of well-chosen stepping stones towards an explanatory or causal conclusion, but a collection of ideas generated by perceived similarities to a number of combined facts observed with the patient. These kind of hypotheses, therefore, are more like the pictures of particular symptom-configurations that the physician has learned in medical school, or, to be more in agreement with certain other studies, has remembered from experience.

From the example of the multi-level general systems model (Engel, 1980), we designed a five-level structure, ranging from the level of the total human body to a detailed description of processes on the cellular level; a structure which enabled us to arrange the hypotheses according to their specification. The distribution of the generated hypotheses across the levels supported our prediction about the ordering of the hypotheses as depicted above. As might be expected a significant trend towards increasing specification of the hypotheses during the work-up could not be detected. This is hardly surprising when one realized that the first and early hypothesis is usually a specified (level V) one because it stems from a memorized pattern.

Hypotheses generation was evidently not the result of thorough deliberation on the collected evidence. It popped up in the doctor's mind triggered by only a (very) few data. Obviously a (very) superficial resemblance suffices to recognize an assumed similarity. It is the basic process of what is called pattern recognition. It is a process of which the doctor is proud. It is his 'flair clinique' which enables him to deliver immediate judgements.

Pattern recognition is a fundamental feature of animals as well as human beings. It is to this extent hardly understood as a procedure. Especially in animal life this alertness of the mind is of crucial importance for survival. A quick recognition can make all the difference in the world between seeing prey or being prey. Presumably, the animal reacts to superficial resemblances.

Although human beings do not live in animal situations, they use pattern-recognition very extensively every day and every hour. Quick recognition of familiar subjects or objects is sometimes necessary to maintain friendly social relationships (by recognizing your friends), or to survive in traffic or other alarming situations. In the world of advertisement pattern-recognition is of utmost importance in attracting attention. To this end signs and signals have simple and straightforward constructions and elementary colours. They are designed to attract attention by means of simple recognition. Words, names, sentences, ideas, etc., are replaced by one sign. The abstract signal often conceals worlds of concrete meanings, philosophies. One of the world's oldest signs is the cross of Christianity: it covers a universe of religious, philosophical, moral and social rules and concepts.

Pattern recognition without the diagnostic procedure contains at least two different features:

  (a) a procedure, a method; and
  (b) as a conveyer of idiosyncratic contents.

ad a)
From our observations it became clear that pattern recognition as a quick method of comparing similarities plays a major role in inductive reasoning. The initial hypothesis generation in a work-up as well as the following hypotheses are based upon precious little data, which can be demonstrated by the

number of hypotheses prerelated symptoms (HPS) in each cycle. It means that almost all inductive hypotheses must stem from memorized symptom-patterns wrapped in singular (diagnostic) names. The recognition of the symptom-pattern is based on the perception of regularities within the presented facts. The Scottish philosopher Hume (1711–1776) indicated that there are countless (apparent) regularities in nature upon which everybody relies in practice. But we cannot know whether these regularities are man-made (preferring regu-larity over chaos) or law-like occurrences in nature.

'If we have experienced a joint occurrence of A and B, or their quick succession, from this observation does not follow that B is a causal relation from A. How many cases of coherence between A and B we have observed, it cannot be a reason for their cohesion in future. Therefore, induction by simple enumeration cannot be a valid way of reasoning' (Russell, 1948).

This conception questions the conditional probability as a 'true' relation between two events. In that case the second event has to be explained as the (degree of) relation to the first one. When we state 'all swans are black except those photographed during a total eclipse of the sun', we may be perfectly right but its explanation of the relation can be quite different from what we think that it is (Popper, 1983).

As mentioned above, we conjecture regularities in the world as a means of swift decision-making and to maintain a state of emotional certainty. Regu-larities allow reliable predictions' reliable predictions give us the confidence to proceed with our actions. We really want to observe regularities. And what we want to observe is what we get. We collect data with an implicit or explicit question in mind; or as Pascal stated: 'prejudice precedes our view, our observation, and will determine what we shall see'. Our observations are submitted to our judgements, ideas, thoughts. As these conceptions are in-tegral parts of ourselves, the observations can only mirror these conceptions. When we want to observe similarities we may find more similarities than probably exist.

Apparent similarity can lead the physician into blind alleys or to erroneous thinking. Especially the initially formulated hypotheses can force, consciously or unconsciously, the doctor in a particular direction of problem-solving. Any readjustment must come from the physician himself, because the collection of data is directed by the hypothesis previously generated. This is unlikely to happen because it would urge the physician to recommit himself. As we have observed, frequently physicians were kept in a quandary because of the chosen direction, escaping from it by simple guessing.

Sometimes pattern recognition works fine, often not. It is our opinion that pattern recognition (and the modelled repetitive variants) is too unstable a method to be relied upon for quality and efficiency in health care.

ad b)
As mentioned above the generation of the hypotheses is mainly based upon superficial resemblance between a memorized symptom-pattern and some symptoms as presented by the patient. However, when we link the memorized

symptom-patterns with the conception of 'chunks', which we did, then these memorized pictures bear a very personal imprint. The recoding procedure 'rephrases' the collected data into the doctor's 'own words', attaching to it a particular abstract name. In clinical medicine this name will almost be a nosological one, the name of a disease. It may be quite possible that the particular name of a disease contains different contents for physician A than for doctor B. The English philosopher Berkeley (1685–1753) argued that the conceptions men frame, while they may be communicated as de-contextualized abstractions, are nevertheless not framed as abstract ideas but rather are always particularized and specific. Given different physicians they may differ markedly not only in their assessments of a particular case but also to a great extent on the contents of the message they convey in abstract terms. In brief, we can state that the routines are directed at particulars and the results are communicated in abstractions. Berkeley sharply realized the non-existence of what he called 'abstract general ideas'. Any 'abstract general idea' indifferently signifies a great number of particular ideas.

Because of the unique codification and standardization of the data (symptoms and symptom-aspects) we were able to test this notion about 'abstract general ideas' (= name of diseases). Each of the bundled perceptions of the data were matched with the (bundles of perception constituting each mind of the) physicians. The agreement among the grouped physician-participants upon the 'symptoms-contents' of a specified diagnosis scored less than 1%, thus verifying Berkeley's prediction. This finding also reinforces the conception about 'chunking' and recoding. It also warns us to be cautious of accepting abstract names as quantifiable entities.

On diagnoses

What is said about the specific contents of hypotheses is, as a consequence of the inductive process, also valid for the diagnoses. In the diagnosis the highest degree of specification (with respect to the particular physician) is reached. It is the particular entity upon which the doctor is accustomed to (re)act. It represents the endpoint of a reasoning process. So we conjectured that this endpoint describes at least two features:

(1) a similarity of the acquired symptoms and signs as close as possible to the memorized picture of the disease; and
(2) a high(est) estimation of the probability of the correctness of the choice, and minimal feelings of (emotional) uncertainty.

With regard to the former feature we designed two factors for the measurement of consistency of the various symptom-patterns among the participating physicians: the *internal consistency factor (I.C.)* and the *external consistency factor (E.C.)*. The I.C. factor measured the coverage of the acquired data with the description of the diagnosis by the doctor that he had just arrived at. We found an overall coverage of approximately 60%. In our opinion, doctors are rather consistent in their data collection related to their own ideas of the disease. We guessed that the – probably empirically founded – variability known to the physician to exist in disease presentation account for this percentage. We can perceive this factor as some sort of intra-doctor (observer) variation.

In contrast, the E.C. factor represents more or less an inter-doctor variation. We compared the descriptions of the memorized pictures of a particular disease entity, as given by the physicians, with each other. Inter-doctor agreement upon the description of memorized symptom-patterns scored rather low. On average 8% of the symptoms, corresponding to a particular disease, was unanimously mentioned within the group of physicians who described this special picture. Obviously, the memorized pictures of diseases among physicians, even for the most characteristic features of a certain disease, are as different as chalk and cheese.

What we said about abstract nomenclature of hypotheses is ipso facto true for the diagnoses. We must certainly be aware, that as long as we use abstract names for diseases without defining their concrete contents, we, as practitioners in clinical medicine, communicate in vague words and conceptions for which any explanation could be valid.

Clinical decision analysts assume physicians to use, implicitly, probability estimates in their diagnostic procedures. They believe that physicians have, on average, a clear notion of the relative frequency of clinical events within a particular population during a specified time-interval (prevalence, incidence). They surmise that physicians follow a special routine in which the chance estimation of a particular diagnostic hypothesis is adjusted by the subsequent collection of data towards an optimal value (utility). We do not subscribe to this assumption, as might have been clear from the previous chapters.

We asked the participants of the study for their probability estimations of prevalence and incidence. The result was an astounding variability in the figures without the slightest connection to real statistics (when available) whatsoever. Most physicians confessed that they never even considered these factors except in epidemic situations. It might be possible that we sampled a special slice of physicians, but, if that is so, then at least 68 physicians in the world scarcely employ estimates during the diagnostic or therapeutic procedures.

Instead, the physicians rely much more on their feelings of (un)certainty in order to come to a decision. The vacillations in their uncertainty estimates clearly followed certain characteristics of the diagnostic procedure, like, pace of questioning, time consumption, the number of generated hypotheses, the number of hypothesis related symptoms, etc. Taken as a whole, on average these estimations slowly crept towards a maximum, which was only fractionally (25%) higher than the starting estimation. Although we cannot assert without doubt that the physician decides in conformity with (elements of the) Satisficing theory, we gathered the strong impression that he did so, including the typical (re)adjustment of the aspiration level to a maximally attainable goal within the given time interval.

Once a diagnosis is arrived at no further testing will be performed. Obviously, this diagnosis is the most satisfying one. It carries the maximum force of belief; it is the verification of a preconceived solution in mind. The diagnosis carries most of the characteristics of inductivism, including the commitment to the chosen solution. No opposing or contradictory evidence can shake the doctor in his conviction. He has committed himself and there is no urge to recommit himself. Questioning the truthfulness of the diagnosis is questioning the trustworthiness of the doctor.

We replayed the videotaped scenarios some 3–5 days later. We urged each doctor to comment on or to reconsider his work-up, including the possibility to review his diagnosis. None of the physicians reappraised the process or the outcomes. Even in the light of new evidence the chosen solution was maintained. Nobody changed or even questioned his judgement.

The personal and subjective characteristics of the diagnosis led to a confusing arrangement of the attributes. In the light of the subjective characteristics of the diagnosis it is hard to establish the accuracy of the outcome of the diagnostic process as a standard to which all the diagnoses can be compared. As we described in Chapter VI we have chosen for consensus of opinion as some kind of standard (despite all the defectiveness of such a standard). Applying this standard to the material less than 50% of the diagnoses were 'accurate'. As this percentage is also to be found in the literature, it may approximate the percentage of accuracy in actual clinical practice. This figure asks for a thorough reconsideration of diagnostics. But above all, it asks for contemplation on physicians' judgements and the specified contents of the abstract clinical nomenclature.

On prognosis and treatment

Deciding on a treatment is a matter of minutes, as became clear from our study. Only one or two minutes suffice for advising, prescribing and explaining on medication, or referring the patient with a hand-written note to a colleague. It looks as if the therapy section is treated in a Cinderella-like way. But, in my opinion, this conclusion is drawn too easily. We conjecture, on experiential and informal grounds, that the process of deciding on treatment starts during the diagnostic part. Although it cannot definitely be proved from our material, we believe that the possibility and availability of (a) particular treatment(s) have a certain influence on the diagnostic decision; gives it a particular direction. The availability of a particular drug can make the doctor decide to stop further inquiry towards a more refined diagnosis because the aviable treatment covers a whole range of related diseases; further specification of diagnosis will not contribute to more optimal therapy (so the doctor believes).

We found some support for the coincidence of diagnostic consensus with conformity on treatment. This gives the impression that the two processes (if there is such a thing as two processes), that of diagnosis and that of treatment, are concurrent. Regardless of the correctness of the diagnosis the treatment is linked to this conclusion. Among other reasons, we prefer to conceive the clinical process as a unity in which partitions are artificial.

However, this conception of the clinical process hides serious drawbacks. It is often assumed that therapy can act as a test to the diagnosis. When diagnosis and therapy are intimately linked, any serious testing will be illusory. It can lead to self-fulfilling prophecy and self-deception. The disappearance of particular symptoms does not necessarily prove the effectiveness of the therapy, while successful treatment does not necessarily prove the correctness of the diagnosis. Unsuccessful treatment does not necessarily exclude a diagnosis from being accurate, and vice versa. Decision theoretical approach to the clinical process starting from the diagnosis, does not fulfil the necessary criteria that are demanded by this theory.

Another impairment in the directional influence on the diagnostic process can be found as a result of the availability of particular treatments. This availability can take various forms: the availability of particular drugs, the vicinity of alternative health care institutions, the presence of laboratory or X-ray departments, the skills of a surgeon, etc. A surgeon, not really capable of performing a particular operation can, unconsciously, be induced to arrive at an inaccurate diagnosis, a diagnosis where he knows he is capable of handling the treatment. It can induce the doctor to abstain from further acquisition of data or searching for alternative explanations to the presented symptoms when a particular symptom-configuration comes within the range of a treatment: a treatment of which the doctor remembers achieving positive results in more or less similar cases. As we stated before (Chapter IV) it can create a situation of therapies looking for diseases, treatments looking for appropriate patients (Garbage Can model; Cohen, March, Olsen, 1975). Obviously, we need a thorough investigation into this matter in order to elicit more details on these serious drawbacks.

As we stated above (Chapter I) treatment can only be validated by comparison to the (natural) course of a disease. As in most cases the (natural) course of a disease is unknown, most treatment is based on personal opinion and preference. It is particularly in this field that decision analysis tries to bring order and standardization. Through the collection of outcomes of the various treatment options (related to a particular disease) and by standardizing these outcomes in a particular standard value (utility), the track towards the outcome with the highest expected utility can be calculated. Within decision theory too many conceptions about the clinical process have been taken for granted. Some of these conceptions have been discussed. Another is the notion of the well-known prognosis of a disease. We stated in Chapter I that no real prognosis can be given without a proper classification of the disease and a subsequent unequivocal classification of the diagnosis into the pertinent class. However, when a proper classification is still lacking and the placing of a correct, uniformly defined, diagnosis into the right class is reached in only half of the cases, proper prognosis is still wanting. Without a proper prognosis most treatment actions remain void of meaning apart from alleviating the suffering. Probabilistic approach to these actions seems to be rather unavailing.

We asked the participating physicians about their knowledge of the prognosis of the disease they had just diagnosed. Apart from some general statements like 'I think the patient will recover' or 'the complete recovery of the patient is dubious', or 'I do not think the patient will survive', any precise prediction about the course of a disease is wanting. As they state, physicians usually rely on their remembrance of courses of similar cases in the recent past. Apart from the unreliability of judgements from memorized events, as was brilliantly demonstrated by Tversky and Kahnemann (1974), the very personal and impressionistic conception of these remembrances cannot contribute to a consistent apprehension of prognosis.

The study of the natural courses of diseases is seriously impaired by the clinical actions. In most cases the course of the disease, whether known or not, is influenced by the medication or other form of therapy prescribed by the doctor. We can see this as a consequence of the health care system. No physician is allowed to stay in the wings in cases of, for instance, pneumonia when penicillin is within reach. Medicine as a social institution cannot afford to withdraw from its first duty: health-care delivery and assistance, alleviation of the sufferings of the patient, to the disadvantage of the other imperative: to strive for a scientific foundation of medical knowledge. Consequently, medicine is trapped by its own tasks. Because of its caring duties it has to renounce its scientific task, while the scientific task is to provide the necessary knowledge to perform that health care adequately.

Unless we are able to learn the prognosis of a particular disease, we cannot know whether any favourable or unfavourable effects must be attributed to the course of the disease, the wishful thinking of the doctor or the patient, or to supernatural forces. Any statement about treatment must, in these cases, be taken with much caution.

On learning and experience

It is widely assumed that we (can) learn from experience. 'Experience is the best teacher' the proverb says. However, what exactly we learn from experience is left to the imagination. Some people even question the assumption. According to Brehmer (1980) one thing may be clear: we certainly do not learn from experience; at least not in the medical world. Several obstacles prevent the physician from learning from his clinical work. The individualistic character of the medical process excludes by its very existence a number of options. When a physician prescribes drug X it excludes the prescription of drug Y for the same patient, otherwise than in combination. Prescription also debars non-prescription. The advantages or disadvantages of drug X for the patient cannot be compared with the advantages or disadvantages of drug Y for the same patient at the same moment. Other patients and other moments create different circumstances.

The judgement of treatment results can be tainted by our expectations. For instance, many patients will differ in opinion from their physicians with regard to the results of a particular treatment: the effects of a dermatological treatment, remaining scars after an operation, etc. Presumably it is not the results but the differing expectations that colour the scene.

Observational errors can also follow from anticipation. For instance, when a doctor does not expect to find cardiac murmurs, he usually finds none; when he expects to palpate an enlarged spleen, he will find it. Seriousness, or presumed seriousness, of illness can be another source of observational error or misjudgement. Presumed urgency can lead the doctor to so-called life-saving interventions, although sometimes a watchful expectation would be more appropriate. Retrospection does not solve the problem. As we argued, inductive reasoning excludes the reversibility of the process. It cannot explain the causes of failures, because the operational principle bears in it the conditions for success. In this sense, the medical process is a one-way process. But when feedback mechanisms do not exist, how can a physician learn from these instances? How can he learn by trial and error when he cannot detect the causes of the errors?

Still, we still possess an intuitive feeling of something to be learnt from experience. Evidently, we prefer the skilled surgeon to the novice; we bypass the dentist who has never yet extracted a tooth; we prefer the skilled labourer to the unskilled. Should we mistrust our feelings (which is often to be recommended) or is there another explanation for the nature of experience? Although the results of our study indicate a lack of effect on improving competence through experience, we shall briefly comment on this subject.

From the example mentioned above we may propose a difference between experience as related to skills, and experience as related to intellectual tasks like problem-solving. Every amateur doing a job, for instance in the house, knows the difference between his efforts as compared to those of the professional. The more we perform a particular action the more we become skilled in its execution. The more we drive a car the more we are accustomed to its mechanism, which contributes to safer driving as the driver can devote all his attention to the traffic. 'Practice makes perfect': the continual practice or repetition of an activity leads to perfection in its performance. In this sense, obviously we can learn from experience.

But, as some people will remark, skills are different from intellectual tasks like problem-solving or decision-making. Unlike performing tasks by hand immediate feedback in intellectual tasks is not always offered. As mentioned above, feedback is a necessary condition for learning from experience. We learn from our errors only when we recognize them as errors and adopt an attitude in which criticism can be accepted as valuable. Apparently, learning from experience requires not only an intellectual challenge but also a particular personal attitude. It asks for people with a particular question in mind and who are open to information. 'Experience' is gained by learning from our mistakes. It is gained by an actively critical approach: by the critical use of experiments and observations designed to help us to find where we have gone astray (Popper, 1983).

It is exactly at this latter point that the inductive reasoning process leaves us empty-handed. Principally, its process cannot be traced back, and its outcome does not unequivocally follow from the acquired evidence, but is based on personal belief. It does not invite 'open-mindedness', the formulation of unsolved questions or a search for alternative answers. Instead, it fosters a closed attitude, an attitude of 'I knew it all along'. Here we do not look for any new solution of a problem, but try to become familiar with the solutions previously discovered by trial and error. In inductive reasoning we observe similarities or take certain positions. Socrates frequently made his partners realize that they held theories or views of which they were not fully aware and which sometimes were even conflicting. But where is the Socrates of our time who will reflect on our reasoning processes and criticize our judgements?

Repetitions create a 'habit', a state of mind in which we are inclined to see resemblances upon which we can act by performing known skills or routines. And even if the resemblance is faint, we appeal to a common origin by explaining it by similarity of a higher order. From this we can create a metaphysical system apt to 'explain' similarities from some higher order which in its turn derive their resemblances from a still higher order, and so on. This metaphysical system makes us observe similarities whether they are real or not. Problems are no longer solved by the act of reasoning but by routine. In that case experience does not contribute to learning, to the acquisition of new knowledge. Instead, it may produce a negative effect; an effect in which even complicated problems are approached by simple routines.

Experience has two faces: a positive one, in which learning as an act of acquiring new knowledge takes place; and a negative face, in which problem-solving is replaced by simple routine, detracting from optimal judgement. As it might be possible that the results of both groups are represented in our material, the outcomes of the matching of 'experience' to a number of variables produced an indeterminate result. As the material is not specific enough on this point we cannot present any definite answer.

From these reflections on experience we come to the conclusion that at least two ways of learning can be recognized. First, learning by trial and error. In order to acquire new (theoretical) knowledge an 'open-minded' attitude is required; it demands the application of an intelligent problem-solving process to the problem, which unsolved, continues to irritate us. Secondly, 'learning' by habit formation, or by repetition. This type of 'learning' can only partially contribute to our competence in solving problems. Popper (1983) recognized a third type: learning by imitation. It is one of the more primitive and important forms of learning. Here the highly complex instinctual basis of learning and the role played in it by suggestion and by the emotions are more obvious than in the other ways of learning. For example, the child discovers how to walk by imitation. From this stage the newly discovered skill is 'practised' until it becomes a habit. In medicine this latter type of learning is a usual feature in teaching. Of old, the apprentice in medicine turned to a master, a well-known example of his profession, and got his lessons by closely watching the skills of his teacher. Nowadays, students go to medical school, get a basis of practical and impractical knowledge, and are placed with a teacher who tells them to scrutinize his, the teacher's, skills and behaviour, and to imitate him. Training for these skills and behaviour can be accomplished on patients placed at the student's disposal by the teacher. Measurement of the clinical competence is accomplished by making a comparison between the knowledge, skills, and behaviour of the students with those of their teacher (or peer group). This type of training does not foster the intellectual challenge of (complicated) problem-solving and an 'open-minded' attitude.

The relationship between learning and experience in clinical practice, therefore, remains troublesome.

On medical research

Although this was not part of the investigation, it is related to it by the inductive versus deductive styles. We can describe the aim of scientific research as the finding of satisfactory (or causal) explanations to whatever puzzles us. What applies to problem-solving can also be ascribed to the processes and methods in (medical) research. We shall briefly comment on this subject.

As mentioned in Chapter II much in medical knowledge is still in need of causal explanation. For the application of the deductive strategy in clinical practice scarcely no suitable domain can be found. Comprehensive and explanatory theories for most (groups of) diseases are still being awaited. For many of the prevalent diseases, like myocardial infarction, arterial diseases, cancer, rheumatological and degenerative diseases, several viral diseases, psychiatric illnesses, definitive answers are still wanting. Medicine has only diffuse ideas about most diseases, and, what is more, these ideas cannot always successfully stand trial by scientific test. Many theories live on despite being proven incorrect ('the mysterious viability of the false').

Nevertheless, most medical research is aimed at the description of single cases, or small groups of patients, by trying to find a common denominator which can explain (a number of) the features of the disease under study. It is the straightforward example of induction by enumeration: from the acquired data some insight into the subject will be obtained (see Chapter II). It is the method of drawing verifying instances from observations, raising these instances to general theories, regardless of whether one is aware or unaware of the fallibility of such reasoning.

The method can be perfectly understood. A special phenomenon attracts the doctor's attention. His curiosity is raised, and he starts looking around for similar phenomena with similar patients. Then he collects as much data from the (small group of similar or assumed similar) patient(s), being careful to stick as closely as possible to the data without interpretation (avoiding bias). He then analyses the collected data with or without the help of (mathematical) statistics (usually *with* statistics because of the demands of several scientific journals) and draws conclusions from high-grade correlations between the observed phenomena and some critical features of the patients. However, as Hume and Russell stated, however many correlations we may find, it only explains the co-existence of two or more phenomena (and their repeated occurrence) without being explanatory of any theory of causal explanation.

For instance, one observes a frequently encountered phenomenon in a population, e.g., hypertension. The investigator defines upper and lower limits of the blood pressure of a sample of patients. He designs a number of variables which may or may not be connected to the hypertension. He then starts with the acquisition of data from the sample, being as strict as possible. Statistical analysis then tells him that a co-occurrence of two or more variables with a certain degree of probability can be detected. However, although hundreds and hundreds of these investigations have been performed, we in medicine still have no notion of the cause or the exact nature of hypertension. Nevertheless, millions of people all over the world are treated for hypertension.

Some institutions are occupied with the mere collection of data for the sake of the data themselves. Investigators can knock at their door for specific data on a particular domain. These data are then analyzed, usually by means of statistical procedures, and the results are extrapolated to the total population and are propagated as the scientific proof demanding a change in management or some type of policy. An independent test of the experimental results is still wanting.

These inductive-style studies are so common, that most people hold them as scientific. Even some scientific journals predominantly publish inductive-style papers, thus corroborating the idea that this style really is scientific and explanatory.

The basic idea of an inductive-style investigation is reliance on observations, on data. One must keep carefully to the actual observations and beware of early theorizing. Theorizing can easily create bias or colour the observations. As these observations are the basis for one's analysis, and from that the basis of a 'general theory', any pollution of the data can be disastrous to the theory and its generality. A paper on an inductive-style investigation, therefore, must scrupulously denote the data, their acquisition, and their analysis in order to be credible. Popper (1983) illuminatingly presents the following structure of an inductive-style paper.

(1) It first explains the preparation for our observations. To these belong, for example, the experimental arrangements, such as the apparatus used, its preparation for the experiment, and the preparation of the objects of observation.

(2) The main part of the paper consists of a theoretically unbiased pure description of the experimental results: the observations made, including measurements (if any).

(3) There follows a report of repetitions of the experiment, with an assessment of the reliability of the results, or of probable errors (lately this may include statistical work).

(4) Optional: a comparison of the results with earlier ones, or with those of other workers in the field.

(5) Also optional: suggestions for future observations, for desirable improvements to the apparatus, and for new measurements.

(6) The paper is concluded (again optionally) by a brief epilogue, usually of a few lines only, and sometimes in a smaller print, containing a formulation of a hypothesis suggested by the experimental results of the paper.

These points are not always rigidly adhered to. Some points may be omitted, others added. What I do suggest is that there is a tendency to make young scientists believe that this is the proper way to present results, and that even masters adhere to this way of presentation (Popper, 1983).

This does not mean that this style of investigation does not have its potential value. It can emphasize the gaps in our knowledge, the absence of causal explanations. It can attract attention to particular problems or problem areas in need of explanation. It can suggest a further scientific research project. It can be a first step in that difficult domain called scientific research. But it cannot replace deductive investigation nor can it be assumed to be the complete version of a scientific study. It is a preliminary study, no more no less. Within this context it bears its own value.

Without a suggestion for a structure of a scientific paper this section could not be complete. Again we shall quote Popper (1983) for his proposal of a standard experimental paper.

(1) A clear exposition of the problem – or, if the problem may be assumed to be well-known, a clear reference to it and to an exposition of it. The author should also make it clear whether he accepts the problem situation as sketched by some predecessor or whether he sees the problem differently. This would give the author an opportunity to clarify for himself (and perhaps for others) the always shifting problem situation.

(2) A more detailed survey of the relevant hypotheses bearing on the problem (and of the experiments bearing on the hypotheses, indicating the degree to which these are able to contribute to the appraisal of the hypotheses).

(3) A more specific statement of the hypothesis (or hypotheses) which the author intends to propose, or to discuss, or to test experimentally.

(4) A description of the experiments and their results.

(5) An evaluation: whether the problem situation has changed; and if so, how.

(6) Suggestions for further work arising from the work reported.

We, in medicine, are in need of causal explanations for an infinite number of diseases and related health care areas. Only through theories or bold statements (based or unbased on observation) can we come nearer to the truth. Only through theories which can be reasoned through to their detailed consequences can we reach explanations and learn causal relationships. For theories constitute the network of co-ordinates for science.

Closing remarks

It was my intention to provide a small contribution to the elucidation of the methodology as it is used in clinical practice, with a special eye on teaching and learning. It resulted in the question whether physicians use a deductive or an inductive method of problem-solving and decision-making. Within the group of sixty-eight physicians-participants the inductive method was exclusively employed. We conjecture from this finding that the inductive type of reasoning is the predominant style in the medical world.

The consequences attaching to the overall utilization of the inductive method are far-reaching. It gives rise to a very personalistic orientation to medicine. It defines 'medicine' as an accumulation of personal conceptions about health and disease instead of being an autonomous, generally applicable, science. Abstract terms conceal variant concrete contents; comparability of concepts, terms, statistics, etc., is barred; outcomes and treatments carry personal preferences instead of being well-founded judgements. Numerical estimations contain highly individualistic perceptions. The inductive method relies on memories of the users; memories prone to the fallibilities of all human thinking processes. By its nature the inductive strategy is irretraceable. Consequently, errors in reasoning cannot be detected. Feedback cannot be provided. Outcomes of inductive reasoning processes are a matter of belief, and, therefore, unquestionable. Besides, these outcomes (diagnoses, treatment plans) are supported by personal commitment which prevents (re)consideration.

But why is inductive reasoning practised on such a world-wide scale? In my opinion it is because induction is the most basic process in thinking and behaviour. It is the method of intuition, of quick (pattern) recognition, of fast action, of survival. It is also the method which allows imagination and fantasy, creative and heuristic steps. It allows emotions and feelings to slip into the reasoning process. It permits the physician to act in a way which he assumes appropriate in human-to-human contact. It is also how the patients want the doctor to behave: a curing but above all a caring person, a trusted and reliable human being, taking care of all those little and great pains, sufferings and sorrows that can beset our lives. In short, it allows for art-like behaviour by the physician.

But I see it as my task to make explicit what is implicit. To show, to make observable the steps and the actions, the thoughts and the deliberations of physicians solving-problems that patients present to them. To assist in recognizing what is going on for the purpose of understanding and improving the processes of caring and curing people. It resulted in the question: 'Is medicine an art or a science?' This unanswerable question was reduced to the more mundane question whether induction is an artistic or scientific method. As is usually the case with such big questions, the answer cannot be conclusive. I have brought together a number of ideas, facts, and conceptions. Should you feel the urge to contemplate further on these ideas, facts, and conceptions, then my objective will have been reached.

REFERENCES

Adlassnig, K.P. (1980): A fuzzy logical model of computer assisted medical diagnosis. *Meth. Inf. Med.* **19**, 141–148.

Albert, D.A. (1978): Decision theory in medicine. *Milbank Memorial Fund Quarterly/Health and Soc.* **56**, 362–401.

Allbut, T.C. (1896): *A system of medicine.* London, Macmillan & Co, Ltd.

Anderson, G., Lerena, C., Davidson, D., and Taylor, T.R. (1976): Practical application of computer assisted decision making in an antenatal clinic – a feasibility study. *Meth. Inf. Med.* **15**, 224–229.

Anderson, J.A. and Boyle, J. A. (1968): Computer diagnosis; statistical aspects. *Brit. Med. Bull.* **24**, 230–235.

Asimov, I. (1976): *Unauthorized murder.* London, Gollancz.

Balla, J.I. (1980): Logical thinking and the diagnostic process. *Meth. Inf. Med.* **19**, 88–92.

Balla, J.I. (1982): The use of critical cues and prior probability in decision-making. *Meth. Inf. Med.* **21**, 9–14.

Bariff, M.L. and Lusk, E.J. (1977): Cognitive and personality tests for the design of management information systems. *Management Science* **23**, 820–829.

Baron, D.N. and Fraser, P.M. (1965): The digital computer in the classification and diagnosis of diseases. *Lancet* **ii**, 1066–1069.

Barrows, H.S. and Bennett, K. (1972): The diagnostic skill of the neurologist. *Arch. Neurol.* **26**, 273–277.

Bayes, T. (1763): An essay towards solving a problem in the doctrine of chances. Studies in the history of probability and statistics. *Phil. Trans Roy. Soc.* **53**, 370–418. Reprinted in *Biometrika*, 1958, **45**, 293–315.

Betaque, D.E. and Gorry, G.A. (1971): Automating judgmental decision making for a serious medical problem. *Management Science* **17**, 421–434.

Biörck, G. (1977): The essence of the clinician's art. *Acta Med. Scand.* **201**, 145–147.

Blois, M.S. (1983): Conceptual issues in computer aided diagnosis and the hierarchical nature of medical knowledge. *J. Med. Phil.* **8**, 29–50.

Blois, M.S. (1980): Clinical judgment and computers. *N. Engl. J. Med.* **303**, 192–197.

Bloor, M. (1976): Bishop Berkeley and the adenotonsillectomy enigma: an exploration of variation in the social construction of medical disposals. *Sociology* **10**, 44–61.

Bolinger, R.E., Ahlers, P. (1975): The science of 'pattern recognition'. *JAMA* **233**, 1289–1290.

Boorse, C. (1977): Health as a theoretical concept. *Philosophy of science* **44**, 542–573.

Boshuizen, H.P.A. and Claessen, H.F.A. (1982): Problems of research into medical problem solving: some remarks on theory and method. *Med. Education* **16**, 81–87.

Bouman, P.J. (1964): *Cultuurgeschiedenis van de twintigste eeuw.* Utrecht, Prisma boeken.

Bower, G. (1967): A Multicomponent theory of the memory trace. In: Spence, K.W. and Taylor Spence, J.T.: *The psychology of learning and motivation.* New York, Acad. Press.

Braithwaite, R.B. (1968): *Scientific explanation. A study of the function of theory, probability and law in science.* Cambridge University Press.

Brehmer, B. (1980): In one word: not from experience. *Acta Psychologica* **45**, 223–241.

Brody, D.S. (1980): The patient's role in clinical decision making. *Ann. Int. med.* **93**, 718–722.

Brown, Hanbury (1986): *The wisdom of science. Its relevance to culture and religion.* Cambridge. Cambridge University Press.

Brunswik, E. (1952): The conceptual framework of psychology. In: *International encyclopedia of unified science* (Vol. 1, No. 10). Chicago, University of Chicago Press.

Brunswik, E. (1955): Representative design and probabilistic theory in a functional psychology. *Psychol. Review* **62**, 193–217.

Card, W.I. (1977): Clinical decision making (1): an analysis. *Health Bull.* 207–212.

Card, W.I. (1970): The diagnostic process. *J. Roy. Coll. Physcns Lond.*, **4**, 183–187.

Carnap, R. (1960): Statistical and inductive probability. In: Madden, E.H. (ed.): *The structure of scientific thought and introduction to philosophy of science.* London, Routledge & Kegan Paul, pp. 269–279.

Carnap, I.R. (1962): The aim of Inductive Logic. In: Nagel, E., Suppes, P., Tarski, A.: *Logic, Methodology and Philosophy of science. Proceedings of the 1960 Intern. Congress Stanford. pp. 303–318.*

Chapman, L.J. and Chapman, J.P. (1967): Genesis of popular but erroneous psychodiagnostic observations. *J. Abnorm. Social Psychology* 72, 192–204.

Cochrane, A.L., Chapman, P.J. and Oldham, P.D. (1951): Observer's errors in taking medical histories. *Lancet* 1007–1009.

Cohen, M.D., March, J.G. and Olsen, J.P. (1975): A Garbage Can Model of Organizational Choice. *Administrative Science Quarterly* 17, 1–25.

Croft, D.J. and Machol, R.E. (1974): Mathematical methods in medical diagnosis. *Ann. Biomed. Eng.* 2, 69–89.

Croft, D.J. (1972): Is computerized diagnosis possible? *Comp. and Biomed. Research* 5, 351–367.

Crookshank, F.G. (1926): Bradshaw lecture on the theory of diagnosis. Part I. *Lancet* 939–942.

Crookshank, F.G. (1926): Bradshaw lecture on the theory of diagnosis. Part II. *Lancet* 995–999.

Cumberbatch, J. and Heaps, H.S. (1976): A disease conscious method for sequential diagnosis by use of disease probabilities without assumption of symptom independence. *Int. J. Biomed. Comp.* 7, 61–76.

Cutler, P. (1979): *Problem solving in clinical medicine.* Baltimore, Williams & Wilkins.

Daal, van, J. (1971): De frequentistische opbouw van de waarschijnlijkheidsrekening volgens R. von Mises. (The frequentistic structure of the probability calculus according to R. von Mises). *Statistica Neerlandica* 25, 117–128.

Dombal, de, F.T., Horrocks, J.C., Walmsley, G. and Wilson, P.D. (1975): Computer aided diagnosis and decision making in the acute abdomen. *J. Roy. Coll. Physcns. Lond.* 9, 211–218.

Dombal, de, F.T. (1978): Medical diagnosis from a clinician's point of view. *Meth. Inf. Med.* 17, 28–35.

Dombal, de, F.T., Horrocks, J.C., Staniland, J.R. and Gill, P.W. (1971): Simulation of clinical diagnosis: a comparative study. *Br. Med. J.* 2, 575–577.

Dombal, de, F.T., Leaper, D.J., Staniland, J.R., McCann, A.P. and Horrocks, J.C. (1972): Computer aided diagnosis of acute abdominal pain. *Br. Med. J.* 2, 9–13.

Dombal, de, F.T., Staniland, J.R. and Clamp, S.E. (1981): Geographical variation in disease presentation. *Med. Dec. Mak.* 1, 59–69.

Dombal, de, F.T. and Gremy, F. (1976): *Decision making and medical care. Can information science help?* Amsterdam, North Holland Publ. Co.

Dornfest, F.D. (1981): The problem solving model of diagnosis in general practice. *South Afr. Med. J.* 59, 298–301.

Dowling, A.F. (1982): Medically oriented computer based information systems. *Med. Care* 20, 253–254.

Driscoll, J.M. and Lanzetta, J.T. (1965): Effects of two sources of uncertainty in decision making. *Psych. reports* 17, 635–648.

Drucker, E. (1974): Hidden values and health care. *Med. Care* 12, 266–273.

Dudley, H.A.F. (1968): Pay-off, heuristics, and pattern recognition in the diagnostic process. *Lancet* 723–726.

Dudley, H.A.F. and Blanchard, E.B. (1976): Comparison of experienced and inexperienced interviewers on objectively scored interview behavior. *J. Clin. Psych.* 32, 690–697.

Eddy, D.M. and Clanton, C.H. (1982): The art of diagnosis: solving the clinicopathological exercise. *N. Eng. J. Med.* 306, 1263–1268.

Einhorn, H.J. and Hogarth, R.M. (1981): Behavioral decision theory: processes of judgment and choice. *Ann. Rev. Psychol.* 32, 53–88.

Einhorn, H.J. and Hogarth, R.M. (1978): Confidence in Judgment: Persistence of the illusion of validity. *Psychological Review* 85, 395–416.

Einhorn, H.J. (1979): Learning from experience and suboptimal rules in decision making. In: Wallsten, T. (ed.): *Cognitive processes in choice and decision behavior.* Hillsdale, N.J., Lawrence Erlbaum.

Elstein, A.S., Kagan, N., Shulman, L.S., Jason, H. and Loupe, M.J. (1972): Methods and theory in the study of medical inquiry. *J. Med. Educ.* **47**, 85–92.

Elstein, A.S., Shulman, L.S. and Sprafka, S. (1978): *Medical Problem Solving*. Cambridge (Mass), Harvard University Press.

Engel, G.L. (1980): The clinical application of the biopsychosocial model. *Am. J. Psychiatry* **137**, 535.

Engelhardt, H.T., Spicker, S.F. and Towers, B. (1979): *Clinical judgment, a critical appraisal*. D. Reidel Publ. Co., Dordrecht, Holland.

Erasmus, D. (1511): *Moriae Encomium (Lof der Zotheid) = Morias egkomion, id est stultiae laus.* (Dutch transl.: Dirkzwager, A.) Rotterdam, Donker, 1986 (Originally published Paris, 1511).

Ericsson, K.A. and Simon, H.A. (1980): Verbal reports as data. *Psych. Review* **87**, 215–251.

Feinstein, A.R. (1977): The haze of Bayes, the aerial palaces of decision analysis and the computerized Ouija Board. *Clin. Pharm. Ther.* **21**, 482–496.

Feinstein, A.R. (1973): An analysis of diagnostic reasoning. 1. The domains and disorders of clinical macrobiology. *Yale J. Bio. Med.* **46**, 212–232.

Feinstein, A.R. (1973): An analysis of diagnostic reasoning. II. The strategy of intermediate decisions. *Yale J. Bio. Med.* **46**, 264–283.

Feinstein, A.R. (1973): An analysis of diagnostic reasoning. III. The construction of clinical algorithms. *Yale J. Bio. Med.* **47**, 5–32.

Feinstein, A.R. (1967): *Clinical judgment*. Baltimore, Williams & Wilkins.

Feinstein, A.R. (1973): The problem of the 'problem-oriented medical record'. *Ann. Intern. Med.* **78**, 751–762.

Fischhoff, B., Slovic, P. and Lichtenstein, S. (1977): Knowing with certainty: the appropriateness of extreme confidence. *J. Exp. Psych. Hum. Perc. Perform.* **3**, 552–564.

Fischhoff, B. (1980): Clinical decision analysis. *Operations Research* **28**, 28–43.

Forstrom, L.A. (1977): The scientific autonomy of clinical medicine. *J. Med. Philos.* **2**, 8–19.

Friedson, E. (1970): *Professional dominance: the social structure of medical care*. New York, Atherton.

Galen (us), C. (1981): *Problems and Prospects*. V. Nutton (ed.), London, Wellcome Institute for the History of Medicine.

Gardiner, R.C. (1978): Quality considerations in medical records abstracting systems. *J. Med. Systems* **2**, 31–43.

Gerritsma, J.G.M. and Smal, J.A. (1982): *De werkwijze van huisarts en internist. Een vergelijkend onderzoek m.b.v. een interactieve patientensimulatie*. Utrecht, W.U. Bunge.

Gill, P.W., Leaper, D.J., Guillou, P.J., Staniland, J.R., Horrocks, J.C. and de Dombal, F.T. (1973): Observer variation in clinical diagnosis. A computer aided assessment of its magnitude and importance in 552 patients with abdominal pain. *Meth. Inf. Med.* **12**, 108–113.

Goldberg, L.R. (1968): Simple Models or Simple Processes? *American Psychologist* **23**, 483–496.

Goldfinger, S.E. (1973): The problem oriented record: a critique from a believer. *N. Eng. J. Med.* **288**, 606–608.

Gorry, G.A. (1974): Modelling the diagnostic process. *J. Med. Educ.* **45**, 293–302.

Griner, P.F., Mayewski, R.J., Mushlin, A.I. and Greenland, P. (1981): Selection and interpretation of diagnostic tests and procedures. Principles and applications. *Ann. Int. Med.* **94**, 553–600.

Groot, de, A.D. (1965): *Thought and choice in chess*. Den Haag, Mouton & Co.

Gross, R. (1977): Was ist eine Krankheit? Gibt es stabile Krankheitsbilder? *Metamed* **1**, 115–122.

Gustafson, D.H., Kestly, J.J., Greist, J.H. and Jensen, N.M. (1971): Initial evaluation of a subjective Bayesian diagnostic system. *Health Serv. Res.* 204–213.

Gutmann Rosenkranz, B. (1976): Causal thinking in erewhon and elsewhere. *J. Med. Phil.* **1**, 372–384.

Harre, R. (1972): *The philosophies of science. An introductory survey*. Oxford, Oxford University Press.

Helfer, R.E. and Slater, C.H. (1971): Measuring the process of solving clinical diagnostic problems. *Br. J. Med. Educ.* **5**, 48–52.

Hippocrates (1950): *The medical works of Hippocrates*. Oxford, Blackwell.

Howell, W.C. and Fleishman, E.A. (eds.) (1982): *Human performance and productivity. Information processing and decision making*. Hillsdale, Erlbaum Associates.

Howell, W.C. (1982): An overview of models, methods, and problems. In: Howell, W.C. and

Fleishman, E.A. (eds.): (1982): *Human performance and productivity. Information processing and decision making*. Hillsdale, Erlbaum Associates.

Hull, F.M. (1972): Diagnostic Pathways in General Practice. *J. Roy. Coll. Gen. Pract.* **22**, 241–257.

Hume, D. (1978): *Het menselijk inzicht (An enquiry concerning human understanding)*. Meppel, Boom.

James, W. (1890): *Principles of psychology*. New York, Holt.

Janis, I.L. and Mann, L. (1977): Emergency decision making: a theoretical analysis of responses to disaster warnings. *J. Human Stress* 35–48.

Janis, I.L. and Mann, L. (1977): *Decision making*. New York, Free Press.

Johnson-Laird, P.N. and Wason, P.C. (1977): *Thinking, readings in cognitive science*. Cambridge University Press.

Kahnemann, D. and Tversky, A. (1972): Subjective probability: a judgment of representativeness. *Cogn. Psych.* **3**, 430–454.

Kahnemann, D. and Tversky, A. (1973): On the psychology of prediction. *Psych. Review* **80**, 237–251.

Kahnemann, D. and Tversky, A. (1979): Prospect Theory: an analysis of decision under risk. *Econometrica* **47**, 263–291.

Kassirer, J.P., Moskowitz, A.J., Lau, J. and Pauker, S.G. (1987): Decision Analysis: A progress report. *Ann. Int. Med.* **106**, 275–291.

Kassirer, J.P. (1976): The principles of clinical decision making: an introduction to decision analysis. *Yale J. Biol. Med.* **49**, 149–164.

Kellert, S.R. (1976): A sociocultural concept of health and illness. *J. Med. Philos.* **1**, 222–228.

Kleinmuntz, B. (1982): Computational and noncomputational clinical information processing by computer. *Behav. Science* **27**, 164–175.

Kleinmuntz, B. (1968): The Processing of clinical information by man and machine. In: *Formal representation of human judgment*. New York, John Wiley & Sons, pp. 149–186.

Kleinmuntz, B. (1963): Profile analysis revisited: a heuristic approach. *J. Couns. Psychol.* **10**, 315–321.

Kleinmuntz, D.N. and Kleinmuntz, B. (1981): Systems simulation. Decision strategies in simulated environments. *Behav. Science* **26**, 294–305.

Knill-Jones, R.P. (1975): The diagnosis of jaundice by the computation of probabilities. *J. Roy. Coll. Physcns. Lond.* **9**, 205–210.

Kochen, M. (1983): How clinicians recall experiences. *Meth. Inf. Med.* **22**, 83–86.

Komaroff, A.L. (1979): The variability and inaccuracy of medical data. *Proceedings I.E.E.E.* **67**, 1196–1207.

Koran, L.M. (1975): The reliability of clinical methods, data and judgments. *N. Eng. J. Med.* **293**, 642–646.

Koran, L.M. (1975): The reliability of clinical methods, data and judgments (second of two parts). *N. Eng. J. Med.* **293**, 695–701.

Korsch, B.M. and Negrete, V.F. (1974): Doctor-patient communication. *Scientific American* **7**, 66–74.

Lahaye, D., Roosels, D. and Viaenne, J. (1978): The value of subjective appreciation in the medical record. I. The evaluation of dyspnoea. *Meth. Inf. Med.* **17**, 100–103.

Lahaye, D., Roosels, D. and Viaenne, J. (1978): The value of subjective appreciation in the medical record. II. The Evaluation of the general condition of the patient. *Meth. Inf. Med.* **17**, 103–105.

Lakatos, I. (ed.) (1968): *The problem of inductive logic*. Amsterdam, N.Holl. Publ. Co.

Lamberts, H. (1982): Incidentie en prevalentie van gezondheidsproblemen in de huisartspraktijk. *Huisarts en Wetenschap* **25**, 401–405.

Leaper, D.J., Gill, P.W., Staniland, J.R., Horrocks, J.C. and de Dombal, F.T. (1973): Clinical diagnostic process: an analysis. *Br. Med. J.* **3**, 569–574.

Ledley, R.S. and Lusted, L.B. (1959): Reasoning foundations of medical diagnosis. Symbolic logic, probability, and value theory aid our understanding of how physicians reason. *Science* **130**, 9–21.

Leede, de E. and Koerts, J.: *A notion of probability: a survey*. Report, Erasmus University Rotterdam.

Lichtenstein, S. (1972): Conditional non-independence of data in a practical Bayesian decision task. *Org. Beh. Human Perform.* **8**, 21–25.

Lichtenstein, S., Slovic, P., Fischhoff, B., Layman, M. and Combs, B. (1978): Judged frequency of lethal events. *J. Exp. Psych.* **4**, 551–578.

Lindblom, C.E. (1980): *The policy-making process.* Englewood Cliffs, N.J., Prentice Hall.

Lindblom, C.E. (1959): The science of 'muddling through'. *Public Administr. Review* **19**, 155–169.

Lindley, D.V. (1975): Probability and medical diagnosis. *J. Roy. Coll. Physcns. Lond.* **9**, 197–204.

Lindley, D.V. (1975): The role of utility in decision making. *J. Roy. Coll. Physcns. Lond.* **9**, 225–230.

Lusted, L.B. (1976): Clinical decision making. In: Dombal, de, F.T. and Gremy, F.: *Decision making and Medical care. Can information science help?* Amsterdam, N.Holland Publ. Co.

Mandler, G. (1967): The psychology of learning and motivation. In: Spence, K.W. and Taylor Spence, J.T.: *The psychology of learning and motivation.* New York, Acad. Press. pp. 327–372.

Mandler, G. (1967): Verbal learning. In: *New directions in psychology III.* New York, Holt.

Mason, E.E. and Bulgren, W.G. (1964): *Computer application in medicine.* Springfield (Ill.), C.C. Thomas.

Mason, R.O. and Mitroff, I.I. (1973): A program for research on management information systems. *Management Science* **19**, 475–485.

McCarthy, W.H. and Gonnella, J.S. (1967): The simulated patient management problem: a technique for evaluating and teaching clinical competence. *Br. J. Med. Educ.* **1**, 348–352.

McCarthy, W.H. (1966): An assessment of the influence of cueing items in objective examinations. *J. Med. Educ.* **41**, 263–266.

McGaghie, W.C. (1980): Medical problem solving: a reanalysis. *J. Med. Educ.* **55**, 912–921.

McGuire, C.H. and Babbott, D. (1967): Simulation technique in the measurement of problem-solving skills. *J. Educ. Measurement* **4**, 1–10.

McGuire, C.H., Solomon, L.M. and Bashook, P.G. (1976): *Construction and use of written simulations.* New York, The Psychological Corporation, Harcourt Brace Jovanovich.

McKenney, J.L. and Keen, P.G.W. (1974): How manager' minds work. *Harvard Bus. Rev.* **52**, 79–90.

McMullin, E. (1979): A clinician's quest for certainty. In: Engelhardt, H.T., Spicker, S.F. and Towers, B.: *Clinical judgment: a critical appraisal.* D. Reidel Publ. Co., Dordrecht, Holland.

McMullin, E. (1983): Diagnosis by computer. *J. Med. Phil.* **8**, 5–27.

Mechanic, D. (1972): General medical practice: some comparisons between the work of primary care physicians in the United States and England and Wales. *Med. Care* **10**, 402–419.

Mechanic, D. (1972): Social psychologic factors affecting presentation of bodily complaints. *New Engl. J. Med.* **286**, 1132–39.

Mechanic, D. (1978): *Medical Sociology.* 2nd ed. New York, Free Press.

Medawar, P. (1975): Scientific method in science and medicine. *Persp. Biol. Med.* 345–352.

Medawar, P.B. (1969): *Induction and intuition in scientific thought.* Methuen & Co., London.

Medin, D.L., Alton, M.W., Edelson, S.M. and Freko, D. (1982): Correlated symptoms and simulated medical classification. *J. Exp. Psych.* **8**, 37–50.

Meehl, P.E. (1954): *Clinical versus statistical prediction: A theoretical analysis and a review of the evidence.* Minneapolis, Univ. of Minnesota Press.

Meehl, P.E. (1977): Specific etiology and other forms of strong influence: some quantitative meanings. *J. Med. Philos.* **2**, 33–53.

Mettes, C.T.C.W. and Pilot, A. (1980): *Over het leren oplossen van natuurwetenschappelijke problemen; een methode voor ontwikkeling en evaluatie van onderwijs.* T.H. Twente, dissertation.

Miller, G.A. (1956): The magical number seven, plus or minus two: some limits on our capacity for processing information. *Psych. Review* **63**, 81–97.

Miller, G.A. (1962): *Psychology: the science of mental life.* New York, Harper & Row.

Mischel, W. (1979): On the interface of cognition and personality: beyond the person-situation debate. *Amer. Psychologist* **34**, 740–754.

Morrell, D.C. (1972): Symptom interpretation in general practice. *J. Roy. Coll. Gen. Pract.* **22**, 297–309.

Munson, R. (1981): Why medicine cannot be a science. *J. Med. Philos.* **6**, 183–208.

Neisser, U. (1967): *Cognitive psychology*. New York, Appleton-Century-Crofts.

Neumann, von J. and Morgenstern, O. (1947): *Theory of games and economic behavior*. Princeton University Press, Princeton.

Newble, D.I. (1976): The evaluation of clinical competence. *Med. J. Aust.* **2,** 180–183.

Newble, D.J., Hoare, J. and Baxter, A. (1982): Patient management problems. Issues of validity. *Medic. Educ.* **16,** 137–142.

Newell, A. and Simon, H.A. (1972): *Human problem solving*. Englewood Cliffs, New Jersey, Prentice Hall.

Newell, A., Shaw, J.C. and Simon, H.A. (1958): Elements of a theory of human problem solving. *Psychol. Review* **65,** 151–166.

Nisbett, R.E. and Wilson, T.D. (1977): Telling more than we can know: Verbal reports on mental processes. *Psych. Review* **84,** 231–259.

Nobrega, F.T., Morrow, G.W., Smoldt, R.K. and Offords, K.P. (1977): Quality assessment in the hypertension: analysis of process and outcome methods. *N. Engl. J. Med.* **296,** 145–148.

Noren, J., Frazier, T., Altman, I. and DeLozier, J. (1980): Ambulatory medical care, A comparison of internists and family-general practitioners. *N. Engl. J. Med.* **302,** 11–16.

Norusis, M.J. and Jacquez, J.A. (1975): Diagnosis. I: Symptom Nonindependence in Mathematical Models for Diagnosis. *Comp. Biomed. Res.* **8,** 156–172.

Norusis, M.J. and Jacquez, J.A. (1975): Diagnosis. II: Diagnostic Models based on attribute clusters: a Proposal and Comparisons, *Comp. Biomed. Res.* **8,** 173–188.

Oskamp, S. (1965): Over-confidence in case-study judgments. *J. Consult. Psychol.* **29,** 261–265.

Palva, J.P. (1974): Measuring clinical problem solving. *Br. J. Med. Educ.,* **8,** 52–56.

Parsons, T. (1951): *The social system*. New York, Free Press.

Pauker, S.G. and Kassirer, J.P. (1980): The threshold approach to clinical decision making. *N. Eng. J. Med.* **302,** 1109–1113.

Pauker, S.G., Szolovits, P. (1977): Analyzing and simulating. Taking the history of the present illness: Context information. *Comp. Ling. Med.* 109–117.

Pauker, S.G., Gorry, G.A., Kassirer, J.P. and Schwartz, W.B. (1976): Towards the simulation of clinical cognition. Taking a present illness by computer. *Am. J. Med.* **60,** 981–996.

Piaget, J. (1977): Intellectual evolution from adolescence to adulthood. In: Johnson-Laird, P.N. and Wason, P.C.: *Thinking, readings in cognitive science*. Cambridge University Press.

Piaget, J. and Inhelder, B. (1973): *Memory and intelligence*. London, Routledge & Kegan Paul.

Pickering, G. (1979): Therapeutics. Art or science? *JAMA* **242,** 649–653.

Pipberger, H.V., Klingeman, J.D. and Cosma, J. (1968): Computer evaluation of statistical properties of clinical information in the differential diagnosis of chest pain. *Meth. Inf. Med.* **7,** 79–92.

Polanyi, M. (1958): *Personal knowledge. Towards a post-critical philosophy*. London, Routledge & Kegan Paul.

Politser, P. (1981): Decision analysis and clinical judgment. *Med. Dec. Mak.* **1,** 361–389.

Popper, K.R. (1983): *Realism and the aim of science*. Ed. by W.W. Bartley III, Totowa, New Jersey, Rowman & Littlefield.

Popper, K.R. (1972): *Objective knowledge*. Oxford, Clarendon.

Popper, K.R. (1959): *The logic of scientific discovery*. London, Hutchison.

Popper, K.R. (1977): On hypotheses. In: Johnson-Laird, P.N, Wason, P.C.: *Thinking, readings in cognitive science*. Cambridge University Press.

Rapoport, A. and Wallsten, T.S. (1972): Individual decision behavior. *Ann. Review. Psychol.* **23,** 131–176.

Raynes, N. (1980): A preliminary study of search procedures and patient management techniques in general practice. *J. Roy. Coll. Gen. Pract.,* **30,** 166–172.

Redlich, F.C. (1976): Editorial reflections on the concepts of health and disease. *J. Med. Philos.* **1,** 269–280.

Ridderikhoff, J. (1985): The paper patient. In: *Decision making in general practice*. Hounslow, Macmillan.

Rimoldi, H.J.A. (1955): A technique for the study of problem solving. *Educ. Psychol. Measurement* **13,** 450–461.

Rogers, W., Ryack, B. and Moeller, G. (1979): Computer aided medical diagnosis: literature review. *Int. J. Biomed. Comp.* **10,** 267–289.

Rossi, P. (1968): *Francis Bacon, from magic to science*. (transl. S. Rabinovitch). London, Routledge & Kegan Paul.

Russell, B. (1975): *History of western philosophy and its connection with political and social circumstances from the earliest time to the present day*. (Dutch translation) Servire, Wassenaar.

Russell, B. (1956): *Logic and knowledge*. London, Routledge & Kegan Paul.

Sadegh-Zadeh, K. (1974): Subjektive Wahrscheinlichkeit und Diagnose. *Meth. Inf. Med.* **13**, 97–102.

Sadegh-Zadeh, K. (1977): Krankheitsbegriffe und nosologische Systeme. *Metamed* **1**, 4–41.

Sadegh-Zadeh, K. (1980): Toward Metamedicine. Editorial. *Metamedicine,* **1**, 3–10.

Sage, A.P. (1981): Behavioral and organizational considerations in the design of information systems and processes for planning and decision support. *IEEE transactions on systems and cybernetics* **11**, 640–678.

Salamon, R., Bernadet, M., Samson, M., Derouesne, C. and Gremy, F. (1976): Bayesian method applied to decision making in neurology – methodological considerations. *Meth. Inf. Med.* **15**, 174–179.

Scadding, J.G. (1967): Diagnosis: the clinician and the computer. *Lancet*, 877–882.

Scadding, J.G. (1972): Viewpoint. The semantics of medical diagnosis. *Biomed. Comp.* **3**, 83–90.

Scandellari, C. and Federspil, G. (1977): La scelta delle ipotesi in clinica. *Med. Secoli* **14**, 161–181.

Scheerer, M. (1963): Problem-solving. The intelligent solution of a problem seems to involve more than trial and error. Experiments show that it often requires a fresh insight based on a sudden shift in the way the problem is viewed. *Scientific American* **208**, 118–128.

Scheff, T.J. (1963): Decision rules, types of error, and their consequences in medical diagnosis. *Behavioral Science* **8**, 97–107.

Scriven, M. (1979): Clinical judgment. In: Engelhardt, H.T., Spicker, S.F. and Towers, B.: *Clinical judgment, a critical appraisal*. D. Reidel Publ. Co., Dordrecht, Holland.

Shortliffe, E.H., Buchanan, B.G. and Feigenbaum, E.A. (1979): Knowledge engineering for medical decision making: a review of computer-based clinical decision aids. *Proceedings I.E.E.E.* **67**, 1207–1224.

Simon, H.A. (1959): Theories on decision-making in economic and behavioral science. *Amer. Econ. Review* **49**, 253–283.

Simon, H.A. and Newell, A. (1971): Human problem solving. The state of the theory in 1970. *Am. Psych.* **26**, 145–159.

Simon, H.A. (1979): Information processing models of cognition. *Ann. Rev. Psych.* **30**, 363–396.

Simon, H.A. (1976): *Administrative behavior. A study of decision-making processes in administrative organization*. New York, Free Press.

Slovic, P., Fischhoff, B. and Lichtenstein, S. (1977): Behavioral decision theory. *Ann. Rev. Psych.* **28**, 1–29.

Slovic, P. and Lichtenstein, S. (1971): Comparison of Bayesian and Regression approach to the study of information processing in judgment. *Org. Beh. Human Perf.* **6**, 649–744.

Slovic, P. (1982): Toward understanding and improving decisions. In: Howell, W.C. and Fleishman, E.A.: *Human performance and productivity: Information processing and decision making*. Hillsdale, Lawrence Erlbaum.

Smedslund, J. (1966): Note on learning, contingency, and clinical experience. *Scandin. J. Psychology* **7**, 265–266.

Smedslund, J. (1963): The concept of correlation in adults. *Scand. J. Psychology* **4**, 165–173.

Smith, D.H. and McWhinney, I.R. (1975): Comparison of the diagnostic methods of family physicians and internists. *J. Med. Educ.* **50**, 264–269.

Sober, E. (1979): The art and science of clinical judgment: an informational approach. In: Engelhardt, H.T. Spicker, S.F. and Towers, B.: *Clinical judgment, a critical appraisal*. D. Reidel Publ. Co., Dordrecht, Holland.

Sokal, R.R. (1974): Classification: purposes, principles, progress, prospects. *Science* **185**, 1115–1123.

Sokal, R.R. (1977): Classifications: purposes, principles, progress, prospects. In: Johnson-Laird, P.N. and Wason, P.C.: *Thinking*. Cambridge University Press, Cambridge.

Spiegelhalter, D.J. and Knill-Jones, R.P. (1984): Statistical knowledge based approaches to clinical decision support system with an application in Gastroenterology. *J. Roy. Statist. Soc.* **147**, 35–77.

Squire, L.R. (1987): *Memory and Brain*, Oxford, Oxford University Press.

Stern, R.B., Knill-Jones, R.P. and Williams, R. (1975): Use of computer program for diagnosing jaundice in district hospitals and specialized liver unit. *Br. Med. J.* **2**, 659–662.

Tamblyn, R. and Barrows, H. (1978): Evaluation trial of the P4 system. McMaster University, *Monograph* **4**, 4/78.

Tamblyn, R. and Barrows, H. (1978): Teaching guide for the P4 system. McMaster University, *Monograph* **5**, 4/78.

Tautu, P. and Wagner, G. (1978): The process of medical diagnosis: routes of mathematical investigations. *Meth. Inf. Med.* **17**, 1–9.

Taylor, T.R., Aitchison, J. and McGirr, E.M. (1971): Doctors as decision makers: a computer assisted study of diagnosis as a cognitive skill. *Br. Med. J.* **3**, 35–40.

Taylor, T.R. (1976): Clinical decision analysis. *Meth. Inf. Med.* **15**, 216–224.

Thorndike, E.L. (1911): *Animal intelligence: experimental studies*. New York, Macmillan.

Tuchman, B.W. (1985): *The march of folly*. Reading, Abacus, Cox & Wyman.

Tversky, A. (1972): Elimination by aspects: A theory of choice. *Psychological Review* **79**, 281–299.

Tversky, A. and Kahnemann, D. (1973): Availability: a heuristic for judging frequency and probability. *Cogn. Psych.* **5**, 207–232.

Tversky, A. and Kahnemann, D. (1974): Judgment under uncertainty: heuristics and biases. Biases in judgment reveal some heuristics of thinking under uncertainty. *Science* **185**, 1124–1131.

Tversky, A. and Kahnemann, D. (1981): The framing of decisions and the psychology of choice. *Science* **211**, 453–458.

Twaddle, A.C. (1982): Sickness and the sickness career: some implications. In: Eisenberg, L. and Kleinman, A.: *The relevance of social science for medicine*. D. Reidel Publ. Co., Dordrecht, Holland.

Vries Robbe, de, P.F. (1978): *Medische besluitvorming, een aanzet tot formele geneeskunde*. dissertation, Groningen.

Wagner, G., Tautu, P. and Wolber, U. (1978): Problems of medical diagnosis. A bibliography. *Meth. Inf. Med.* **17**, 55–74.

Wagner, G. (1964): Fehlerforschung als Aufgabe der Medizinischen Dokumentation. *Meth. Inf. Med.* **3**, 93–94.

Wason, P.C. and Johnson-Laird, P.N. (1972): *Psychology of Reasoning; Structure and Content*. Cambridge(MA), Harvard University Press.

Weed, L.L. (1970): *Medical records, medical education, and patient care. The problem oriented record as a basic tool*. Chicago, Year Book Med. Pub. Inc.

Werf, v.d., G.Th. (1984): *Geneeskundige Oordeelsvorming*. Amsterdam, Rodopi.

Whitbeck, C. and Brooks, R. (1983): Criteria for evaluating a computer aid to clinical reasoning. *J. Med. Phil.* **8**, 51–65.

Whitbeck, C. (1981): What is diagnosis? Some critical reflections. *Metamedicine* **2**, 319–30.

Wortman, P.M. (1972): Medical diagnosis: an information processing approach. *Comp. Biomed. Research* **5**, 315–328.

Wortman, P.M. and Greenberg, L.D. (1971): Coding, recoding and decoding of hierarchical information in long-term memory. *J. Verbal Learning and Verbal Behaviour* **10**, 234–243.

Wulff, H.R. (1976): *Rational diagnosis and treatment*. Blackwell Scientific Publ., Oxford, London.

Yerushalmy, J. and Palmer, C.E. (1959): On the methodology of the investigation of etiologic factors in chronic diseases. *J. Chron. Disease* **10**, 27–40.

Young, D.W. (1982): A survey of decision aids for clinicians. *Br. Med. J.* **285**, 1332–1336.

Zieve, L. (1966): Misinterpretations and abuse of laboratory tests by clinicians. *Ann. N. Y. Academy of Sciences* **134**, 563–572.

Zola, I.K. (1963): Problems of communication, diagnosis, and patient care: the interplay of patient, physician and clinic organization. *J. Med. Educ.* **38**, 829–38.

Author Index